PRAISE
THE FIVE TIBETANS

C000233158

"It takes vision, courage and the dedication of a true ... *rse
she could have taken in her hometown, so I knew Su* ... *rat
I didn't know was that my willing student was to become my wise teacher. I am so grateful* ... *for
shining her unique light on the Five Tibetan teachings in a way that will inspire people worldwide to
try these fabulous techniques and find their lives changed in positive, meaningful and significant ways.
This work is important and Susan has made it accessible to everyone in this inspiring, authentic and
compelling tapestry of personal stories, clear instruction and insightful wisdom that I am eager to use in
all my Five Tibetan classes from now on."*

— *ELIZABETH HARLEY*, (Meramma Naia), Burghead, Scotland – Reiki Master Teacher, Ascension
   therapist, Five Tibetans Yoga teacher, Master Teacher of the Diana Cooper's School

*"Discovering the Five Tibetans and contemplating the corresponding mantras helped me to acknowl-
edge and release negative patterns of thought and behavior. This book is an enjoyable and practical
guide to some very lofty ideals, and provides a guided path to personal growth and transformation."*

— *CATHERINE DOWD*, 200 RYT – Writer, Yoga Instructor, and Perpetual Student

*"I was fortunate to find out about this program a few weeks after it began. This meant I had to be okay
with being behind on the info and behind on the practice! I've done a lot of yoga in the past, yet this
approach found me at a time in my life when I was ready for its simplicity and gentleness. I have been
amazed that inside of these simple 5 postures I have discovered some new possibilities for myself. The
postures alone don't get the credit, however. It's the simple focus on things such as "vulnerability" and
"surrender". For anyone who wishes to have a deep, yet simple experience of themselves, a cleansing
one, without extra hoopla, I'd recommend getting this book right away. Perhaps the power of this is the
author's own vulnerability and surrender. I'm grateful to have been guided to it."*

— *ROBIN HOLLAND*, CEO Robin Holland International

*"The Five Tibetans Yoga Workshop provided a daily practice of discipline and meditation. The self-
focus time allowed me to sit with my own contemplations and ponderings about subjects that were part
of the content of the workshop. The exercise of the actual Five Tibetans provided physical discipline,
and the mantras of each pose helped me expand my awareness of the impact on my body, mind, and
spirit. I found the work to be profoundly intimate, calming, soothing, and deeply satisfying. Anyone
who has an opportunity to read this book and/or participate in the workshop would be treating themselves to a hugely beneficial experience."*

— *MARGO E. BEBINGER*, CPCC, Leadership and Life Coach, Bigger Game Trainer, Akashic Records
   Practitioner

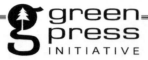

green press

I N I T I A T I V E

Findhorn Press is committed to preserving ancient forests and natural resources. We elected to print this title on 30% post consumer recycled paper, processed chlorine free. As a result, for this printing, we have saved:

4 Trees (40' tall and 6-8" diameter)
2 Million BTUs of Total Energy
396 Pounds of Greenhouse Gases
2,150 Gallons of Wastewater
144 Pounds of Solid Waste

Findhorn Press made this paper choice because our printer, Thomson-Shore, Inc., is a member of Green Press Initiative, a nonprofit program dedicated to supporting authors, publishers, and suppliers in their efforts to reduce their use of fiber obtained from endangered forests.

For more information, visit www.greenpressinitiative.org

Environmental impact estimates were made using the Environmental Defense Paper Calculator. For more information visit: www.papercalculator.org.

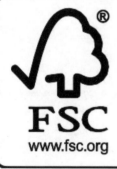

MIX

Paper from responsible sources

www.fsc.org

FSC® C013483

THE FIVE TIBETANS YOGA WORKSHOP

Tone Your Body and Transform Your Life

Susan L. Westbrook, Ph.D.

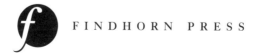

FINDHORN PRESS

© Susan L. Westbrook, Ph.D., 2014

The right of Susan L. Westbrook to be identified as
the author of this work has been asserted by her in accordance
with the Copyright, Designs and Patents Act 1998.

Published in 2014 by Findhorn Press, Scotland

ISBN 978-1-84409-197-3

All rights reserved.

The contents of this book may not be reproduced in any form,
except for short extracts for quotation or review,
without the written permission of the publisher.

A CIP record for this title is available from the British Library.

Edited by Nicky Leach
Cover design by Richard Crookes
Illustrations by Ben Harley
Interior design by Damian Keenan
Printed in the USA

Published by

Findhorn Press

117-121 High Street,

Forres IV36 1AB,

Scotland, UK

t +44 (0)1309 690582

f +44 (0)131 777 2711

e info@findhornpress.com

www.findhornpress.com

To Jenny and Aaron

*Your persistence and amazing
resilience inspire me!*

DISCLAIMER

The information in this book is given in good faith and is not intended to serve as a substitute for informed medical advice or care. As with all forms of physical exertion, if you have any major health concerns, you should first contact your health professional for medical advice and treatment before you start performing these exercises. Neither author nor publisher can be held liable by any person for any loss or damage whatsoever which may arise from the use of this book or any of the information therein.

Contents

Gratitude

The first lesson I learned on the path to this book is that such a venture takes a village—or an army. There may be one name on the cover, but many people contributed to the process. For a leap such as this, I needed nurture, encouragement, money, housing, and consultants for writing and yoga practice. My gratitude to the people who helped bring the book from a vision on a bench at the Berkeley Marina to the manifestation you now hold.

To Laura and my father, who funded the two adventures in Scotland and provided the foundation for this book.

To Alice, Vivian, and Elena, who lived with me and supported me in the "year of my discontent" while the book was coming to life within me.

To my beloved Reiki Master/Teacher Meramma Naia, who gave me the gift of the Five Tibetans one afternoon on the floor of her sitting room in Burghead, Scotland.

To Deborah, Lianne, Gordon, John and Alison, Caroline, and my mother, for providing housing at various times in the process.

To Linda, Freya, Maggie, Nick, Bibi, Amy, Caroline, and Meramma – as readers of the earliest writings you helped me gain the courage and desire to move forward.

To the people in the Findhorn community who offered me friendship and connection.

To my writing coach, Harula Ladd – your guidance in the beginning and the connection you arranged with Sabine created the foundation for the success of the project.

To my editor, Sabine Weeke – thank you for seeing the potential in that rudimentary proposal and for trusting me with the project.

To the original Five Tibetans Workshop group at the Lauvitel Lodge in La Danchere, Venosc, France: Caroline, Maggie, Nick, Pat, and Peter – thank you for your love and commitment. You helped bring the Five Tibetans to life.

To Paula and Hillsborough (NC) Yoga and Healing Arts – thank you for providing space and advertisement for the Five Tibetans Workshop Preview in the US.

To the final reading group: Bibi, Maggie, Nick, and Catherine – thank you for being my support system at the end. You read chapters for a month, stayed with me, and gave me a sense of connection and continuity while so many things were shifting under me. Thank you for your pure expression of friendship.

To Catherine Dowd – you were not only the yoga consultant but also took on the job of chief editor at the end. Thank you for your commitment to excellence.

To Laura and Beth – thank you for your tireless work to create the website platform for me and the book.

I am sure there are others. It has been such an amazing leap. Thank you all for your parts.

Introduction

I was a few days shy of turning 50 years old. I had just climbed 35 feet of ladder and tree studs up a giant California redwood and had hoisted myself onto a platform about two feet square. I lay there, sprawled across the tiny wooden deck like a bear splayed over a tree limb—my legs spread apart and my arms grabbing hold of the far edges of my refuge. I spent several seconds catching my breath and willing myself to crawl to my feet, grateful that the redwood was there to hold onto. Ahead of me was a walk along an eight-foot-long, two-by-six plank suspended in thin air. I knew that once I had conquered that challenge, I would be jumping into space, trying to grab a tiny triangle hanging several meters away. My reward? A fall of more than 30 feet, with nothing to trust in but the harness and four of my peers on the other end of the belay ropes.

I think back to that moment and wonder what I was thinking. Or if I was thinking. I know I was petrified. My heart was beating out of my chest. My limbs were frozen to the platform, my face pressed tightly against the cool wooden surface. My friends were looking on from below, championing my rise from my prostrate pose. I wanted to complete the challenge. I would have also settled for being saved by some unseen force and taken gently back down to the ground. While my faith was great, I figured such an immaculate rescue was not a viable option.

Challenge courses provide out-of-the-ordinary circumstances to allow participants to experience extraordinary parts of themselves. These challenges in the trees also model real life. Hard climbs and long falls. Fear and self-doubt. Acts of courage while the people we love look on in awe and sometimes horror. Inspiration and devastation. Failure and success.

I ultimately got up, hugged the tree, walked the plank, and leapt. The event is aptly named the Lion's Leap. I was met by my friends who gently helped put my feet onto the soft, needle-covered floor of the redwood forest and disconnected my harness from the belay ropes. In that moment there was relief and exhaustion and a welling of tears. I had done it. I had jumped. I had trusted. I had been caught.

I did not know then how closely those moments were going to script the next several years of my life. Originally, a classroom science teacher, university professor, and charter school developer and director, I took a leap out of the mainstream and became a life coach and a high ropes facilitator in 2006. There have been many breath-taking moments since. I lived and worked in France for three years. I hiked with and taught children in the hills of Northern California. I saw my grandson in the first second of his life in this world.

There were also attention-getting moments. Dissolution of relationships. An affair. Persistent unemployment. The illness and death of a long-time friend. Financial instability. Homelessness. I say "attention-getting" because each of those events required something in me that was either lying dormant or lacking altogether. Audacious authenticity. Valuing myself beyond some artificial monetary mark. Letting go of anger and resentment. Not attaching in relationships. Looking deeply within myself, my motivations, and my habits for the ragged edges that needed smoothing and the little dark spots that needed washing away. I had lived a half-century, had helped numerous children and teachers find their way. Now, it seemed, it was time to shine the light on my own darkest corners.

On the platform of the Lion's Leap, as in every high challenge course event, the most important step is the first one. That first step leads you to the second and third, and so on. The first step is where you give yourself full permission to be absolutely terrified—and do it anyway. I find real life to be this way, too. You say to yourself, "This is crazy." Your friends and family may say the same thing. You wonder if you are up to it. Can I really make *that* leap? What happens if I fall?

For me, one of those real-life first steps was following guidance I received in a meditation. I was to seek a teacher and be trained as a Reiki Master. I had no money or real job or place to live at the time I received that message. I took a walk out on the plank of faith and one beautiful fall day in 2011, I packed my 65-liter knapsack, got on a plane, and went to Scotland to begin an intensive apprenticeship with a woman I had never met in a place I had never heard of.

My (now beloved) teacher, Meramma Naia, lived in the little seaside village of Burghead, a few miles from the mystical intentional community known as Findhorn. In addition to our work with Reiki, she offered me instruction in the "Five Tibetans," a legendary set of yoga-like postures touted as the "ancient secret of the fountain of youth" and ascribed with powers of everything from balancing the chakras to setting back the hands of time. I learned the Five Tibetans on the floor of her sitting room, just across the road from the rolling tides and bottlenose dolphins of the North Sea. I practiced the postures every day in the early morning darkness of my little room at the Savitri, a B & B in Findhorn Park.

The Five Tibetans has a world-wide following. If you do an internet search for "Five Tibetans," hundreds of videos, websites, and commentaries will pop up. Evidently, even Dr. Oz does the Five Tibetans! The focus of a majority of those productions is exercise, a perfectly reasonable aspiration considering the number of positive health effects that have been linked to a regular practice of the Five Tibetans. I am now more comprehensively fit than I was when I worked out at the gym three times a week. Participants in our Five Tibetans Workshops have reported significant physical benefits, including reduction in chronic back pain, increased balance, and relief from asthma symptoms. Several pages of similar testimonials occur at the start of Peter Kelder's book, *The Ancient Secrets of the Fountain of Youth*. There is no doubt that regular practice of these five postures can enhance the physical body.

Over time, however, I discovered that the "mystery" of the Five Tibetans was not in doing repetitions of each posture every day; rather, the transformative power lay in the mantras and contemplations originally taught to me by my Teacher and, more recently, the ones I reconstructed for my own practice.

When I began participating in Hatha yoga classes while writing this book, my teacher told us that her yogi had said, "Yoga without breathing is just gymnastics." I immediately understood that statement's parallel with the Five Tibetans: *The Five Tibetans without meditation is just exercise*. While the exercise will be good for your body, the meditative practice can change your life.

Meeting Nonattachment and Nonpermanence

My time in Scotland also led me to consider other ways of thinking about what I expect from life and the stories I tell myself about my past. My teacher had learned the Five Tibetans from Dekyi-Lee Oldershaw, a former Buddhist nun who had studied with a Tibetan Buddhist Master. As I received the poses from my teacher, I was also taught corresponding elements and chakras, as well as the delusions that cause suffering. This was my first substantive exposure to Buddhist philosophy.

Upon my return to the United States, I began to read the works of the venerable Vietnamese Buddhist monk Thich Nhat Hanh. Just as the Five Tibetans became my daily meditation partners, Hanh's book *You Are Here* became the voice that directed my inward steps in those first months after returning from Scotland. I read the little yellow paper back from cover to cover at least four times in the year that followed. It became the symbolic artifact of my year as a spiritual "wanderer."

Although I was unaware of it in the beginning, I was in desperate need of hearing the things Hanh offered in his compassionate yet direct way. Many of the concepts from *You Are Here* will filter into this book. I took the guidance from this gentle monk in the same way I take just about any lesson: I went kicking and screaming. But I also listened. I considered how different the concepts he laid before me were from my own world view. I heard the possibility that things manifest when the conditions are right and do not manifest when the conditions are not right. I learned how to be with my pain as though it were my own precious infant and to believe that the "garbage" of my life can be the "compost" that nourishes the next remarkable part of my path. I worked to extinguish a way of thinking that caused me to see some parts of myself as "bad" and other parts as "good." I am still processing.

Likely, the biggest "Aha!" on that spiritual journey in Buddhist literature was the all-too-obvious reality that everything changes. Nothing is permanent. I am guaranteed nothing—not even my next breath. I know this at some level but tend to try to ignore the truth of it. Once I got my head around the concept of *nonpermanence*, I was hit square on with the accompanying reality of its close partner, *nonattachment.* Simply put, not only can I not expect anything to stay the way it is but I cannot hold onto anything, either. It was a spiritual one-two punch straight to the solar plexus. It took my breath away and shook my sense of security.

I don't know about you, but I believe nonpermanence and nonattachment have to be the hardest concepts of reality we mortals are forced to accept. I want my relationships to last forever. I don't want my friends to die. I don't want to move time and time again. I not only expect things to stay the same but I am shaken to my very core when they do not. Over time, though, I have accepted change as a necessity. I am finding it easier to open my hands and heart to let things go with less grasping and misery. I am not yet an expert at it, but I am more aware of the times I am resisting the flow of "what is."

In many ways, the concepts of nonpermanence and nonattachment are the real teachers in this book. As you read through the chapters that follow, I invite you to explore these realities, both in the world around you and within your own heart and life. Each metaphor from nature or story of my own personal resistance has a built-in connection to the need to accept change and let go of the things and ideas that keep us separated from our best selves and our highest service. Linked with the physical activity of the Five Tibetans and the meditations on the mantras, your ongoing contemplations of nonpermanence and nonattachment will bring about a shift in your expectations which, in turn, will be accompanied by a modification in your thoughts and actions. When you are willing to shift your thinking and your actions, healing and transformation can come streaming in like morning light through an east-facing window.

The purpose of this book is to support your courageous acts of looking deeply and mindfully at the actions and attitudes that create pain in your life, and to coach you forward on the path of living more fully with increased gratitude and joy. The stage for that important work will be a daily practice of the Five Tibetan yogas and contemplation of the accompanying chakras and mantras.

I have titled the book a "workshop" because it is my desire that you will see this as a safe place to tinker with, repair, and build . . . you. Each time you go into the book to read a chapter, visualize yourself walking out the back door of an old farmhouse and heading for the quiet confines of the little workshop down by the pasture. Go in, close the door, gather your tools, and unpack your personality wares and past mistakes. Take stock of your relationship to the concepts of nonpermanence and nonattachment. Take time to consider your attachments. Commit yourself to the work of your own healing and wholeness. I feel confident that when you leave the workshop, you will be well on your way to transforming the behaviors and concepts that are not serving you, and ready to take on ways of thinking and being that can set you free to enjoy a life of intimacy and connection as well as expansiveness and authenticity.

The book is divided into three parts. In Part I, you will get "outfitted" for the journey ahead. You will learn about the Five Tibetan yogas, explore descriptions of the chakras and elements that will be part of the mantras, and get a brief introduction to the stars of the show, i.e., the grasping and healing behaviors. In Part II, you will be led through the five grasping behaviors and their connections to the Five Tibetans and to your life and relationships. In these chapters, you will be asked to explore the ways confusion, resentment, doubt, fear, and miserliness are impacting the choices you make and the life you are constructing. Each of the five chapters will begin with a story taken from a natural setting or my own experience, as a way to create a metaphor for you to carry out of the "workshop" and to use for greater awareness in your daily life. Part III offers the antidotes to the grasping behaviors—actions that can bring healing and wholeness and a greater sense of connection to yourself and to the world. As you complete the journey, you will be encouraged to contemplate the impact your commitment to awareness, vulnerability, surrender, authenticity, and connection can have on your sense of self and on your relationships.

In essence, this book is a spiritual workshop between two covers. When I say the word "work," my mind automatically hears my young grandson, Ben, say, "I have wuk to do!" I assume he hears that from his parents, but the sweet chirp of his voice and his toddler's semi-lisp make it an irresistible statement. I find myself repeating it, adding the rise in pitch on the word, "wuk" as he does. There *is* work to do. To heal the results of the hurts and disappointments that have come your way. To open your heart to greater love and compassion for yourself and others. To create a confidence and peace that will allow you to stride out into your world and your relationships with greater joy. Yes, there will be some ease and flow. Yes, there is also work to do. It is a courageous act; there is no harder job on the planet than standing steady and taking a look inside at all those layers we have constructed over the years. You are here today because you believe it is time to do that work. You have been led to this perfect place at this perfect time for your perfect healing. Welcome to your workshop!

Part I
Preparing

The Journey Begins

It was not quite 7 o'clock on a mid-September Sunday morning in the East Bay. I rode my bicycle from the apartment, along the designated bike route, and down to the Berkeley Marina. As it was still early, I was one of only a few people in a place that would soon become crowded with walkers and animal lovers, cyclists and kite flyers. I coasted to a familiar spot directly across the bay from the Golden Gate Bridge. The air was crisp, the sky blue, and the water choppy in the ever-present wind coming over from the Pacific Ocean.

I was there on this day to ponder what was to become of me. My live-in relationship had just ended abruptly. Out of work and with no prospects to support myself immediately, I had been forced to ask my father for money for the first time in my adult life. I had no idea where I was going or what I would be doing.

I approached the two benches in front of me, looking first to the one on the left where I usually sat meditating, views of the water, San Francisco, the bridge, and the "hills" of Sausalito before me. But this day, I turned and moved toward the bench to my right. As I took off my helmet and settled down on the wooden surface beaded with condensation from the morning fog, I noticed a brass plate in the center of the back of the bench. Printed on a plaque dedicated to a woman named Harriet Shaffer was a quote attributed to Helen Keller:

"Security is mostly a superstition.
It does not exist in nature.
Life is a daring adventure, or nothing."

I sat on that bench that morning and cried and wrote and prayed. By the time I got back on my bike to cycle to the house that would no longer be my home, I knew what I was going to do. The message had been clear. Write the book. I would be going back to Scotland, back to my teacher and the people I had met a year earlier, to write the book I had intended to write in the year I had been in Berkeley—a book that lived in my heart, but like a too-large shard of glass had just not made its way out of me and onto pages.

Thirty minutes later, I arrived at the apartment. I walked in the door and said, "I am going to Scotland to write my book." I felt immense freedom and possibility. There was an adventure before me! I held my arms out to allow my wings to unfold and felt the soaring begin.

CHAPTER 1

The Five Tibetan Yogas

W hile writing this book, I had the opportunity to do a Five Tibetans Workshop at a yoga studio in North Carolina. As we gathered in the building's foyer, a man entered, looked around, and asked where the "five Tibetans" were. It became something of a joke as the afternoon went along. He had, perhaps, expected to find five monastic monks in their robes and regalia ready to teach him yoga. Instead he found me: a middle-aged woman in black stretch pants and a T-shirt. While this story will later be expanded to include a tale of stage fright and smallness, for the present it serves to introduce the namesake of our workshop. The Five Tibetans are not a "who"; they are a "what."

The Five Tibetans are legendary yoga-like postures that were reportedly part of the daily practice of monastic monks in Tibet, who performed the five exercises to balance the energy of the chakras and to enhance vigor and vitality. The history of the Five Tibetans is as much lore as it is truth.

In 1939, an American by the name of Peter Kelder published a small book called *The Eye of Revelation* (later re-released as *The Ancient Secret of the Fountain of Youth*), in which he gave accounts of his experiences with a retired British army officer he referred to as Colonel Bradford. Colonel Bradford, as the story goes, had been a physically debilitated man in his sixties when he had disappeared with his walking cane into the wilds of Tibet searching for what he had been told was the ancient fountain of youth. I appreciated Kelder's assessment of Colonel Bradford's physical status at that time: "Like so many other men, Colonel Bradford had become old at the age of 40 and had not grown any younger."

As Kelder spins the tale about the colonel's discovery of a set of exercises he called "The Rites of Rejuvenation," we are led to believe that doing the five exercises on a daily basis can, quite literally, set back the aging process. Whether these five exercises or rites or yoga postures originated in a Tibetan monastery or not, they are now practiced by people all over the world. In this chapter you will learn the basic poses of the Five Tibetans and ways to make them the core of your daily personal practice. I imagine you will have questions about particulars as you read through this chapter. If so, I invite you to visit the Five Tibetans Workshop website (*www.5tibetansworkshop.com*), where you will find videos, information, and a blog designed to help you as you move along on your journey.

Please remember, as with all forms of physical exertion, if you have any major health concerns, you should not perform these yogas without first securing the advice of your medical/holistic practitioner.

The Five Tibetans and Hatha Yoga

I will refer to the Five Tibetans as yoga poses in this book; however, they differ from the yoga you may have done in yoga studios in several ways. First, the Five Tibetans do not have names; they are simply called First, Second, and so on. You may recognize aspects of the poses you performed in yoga class in the Five Tibetans, but I will primarily refer to them by their numbers.

The second practical difference between the Five Tibetans and Hatha yoga is that rather than holding a pose for an extended time, Tibetans Two to Five are performed as a series of rhythmic repetitions. The First Tibetan, as you will see, is an outlier of sorts but is still executed as a set of repetitions. Newcomers to the Five Tibetans generally begin with three repetitions of each of the poses. As you continue your practice, you will add repetitions until you reach the suggested number of 21. The length of time you hold a pose will depend on your personal goals.

The third distinction between the Five Tibetans and Hatha yoga is found in the timing of the inhalations and exhalations of the breath. In each repetition of a Five Tibetan posture, you will inhale as you "fold" and exhale as you relax back into the start position. This pattern of breathing is opposite to that of Hatha yoga, where the exhalation occurs on the "fold." In her book *Chakra Workout: Balancing the Chakras with Yoga*, Mary Horsley proposes that the reason for this shift in the pattern of the breath "concentrates the energy in the Sushumna, the body's principal *nadi*, or meridian, which connects all the chakras" (p.124). This explanation is plausible, given that balancing the chakras and increasing the speed of their spins was the reason Colonel Bradford gave for the monks' performance of the Five Tibetan "rites" in the monasteries.

I want to make a request at this point in our relationship: that you do not approach the Five Tibetans as an exercise program. I ask that, because I, as a former gym enthusiast, understand that exercise programs may have a different focus and culture than seem fitting for the Five Tibetans. Exercise programs can spur feelings of competitiveness and self-aggrandizement. When you take on a daily practice of the Five Tibetans, you are not in competition with yourself or anyone else. The practice is not meant to be about seeing how many repetitions can be done in how little time.

Performing the Five Tibetans, as with any yoga, is about a balance of mind and body and spirit. I consider my daily experience with the poses to be sacred. My mat, then, is a sacred space where I treat the Five Tibetans like my closest friends and confidants. They have been with me during difficult and growth-producing times. I guarantee if you stick with them, you will feel your body increase in strength and stamina. And I encourage you to allow the process to proceed gently, from a place of spirit and balance and love.

The Rest Poses

Between each set of each of the Five Tibetans you will move into a rest pose. The purpose of the rest pose is to regain the rhythm of your breath and to meditate on the mantra. In Hatha yoga, these are known as restorative poses. I will speak more about the rest poses as we move onward in the journey, but will include a short description of each one here.

The First, Third, and Fifth Tibetans are followed by the Hatha yoga pose known as Child's Pose. In Child's Pose, you kneel on the mat, sit back on your feet, and bend your torso over so that your chest is on your thighs or on the mat. You may choose to put your feet together and spread your knees toward the edges of the mat or to hold your legs parallel to one another.

When you first bend into the pose, put your arms out in front of your head and feel the stretch in your back and shoulders. When you are ready, pull your arms back along the sides of your body and let your forehead rest on the mat. You may rest your head on a pillow or a yoga block if your head does not easily reach the floor. Allow your hands to relax and your palms to face upward.

Breathe deeply as you hold this pose. Notice your breathing and remain in the pose until your breath has become relaxed and rhythmic. As the parasympathetic nervous system kicks in, you may experience a slight sigh or shudder signaling that you have, indeed, achieved a state of relaxation.

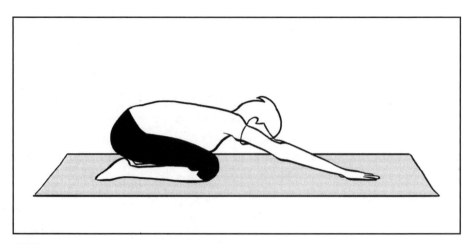

Child's Pose

After the Second and Fourth Tibetans, you will rest in Corpse Pose. Lie on your back on the mat with your legs straight out and your feet 8–10 inches apart and relaxed, allowing the legs to roll open naturally. Your feet should be wide enough apart that your lower back releases. Your arms rest at your sides, palms up, hands a few inches from your body. If you have any discomfort in your back, place a bolster or a rolled blanket under your knees. Breathe deeply and rhythmically. The purpose of this pose in traditional yoga is to allow time and opportunity for renewal and rebirth, usually at the end of a yoga session. In the chapters that follow, I will encourage you to use this pose as a way to clear away any remaining thoughts or emotions that are not serving you.

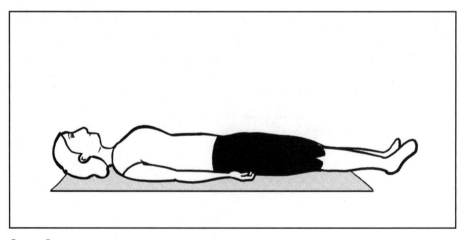

Corpse Pose

Corpse Pose is also an excellent pose in which to consciously practice taking and releasing a complete breath. To do this, draw in air through your nose while contracting down on your diaphragm, the muscular dome-shaped plate right beneath your ribcage. You will feel your lungs fill with air as your belly inflates in size. You can try that right now, as you sit here reading. Being a "belly conscious" society, we have a tendency to want to suck in our stomachs rather than to allow them to protrude. In order to breathe completely, you will need to permit yourself to let your belly become soft and large when you take in the breath. As your belly continues to enlarge, let the breath rise to expand your ribcage up and out to the sides. Finally, allow the breath to come up into your upper chest and throat. Now exhale by relaxing and allowing the breath to exit, leaving the belly flat and the ribcage contracted.

As you practice taking complete breaths, you may want to think of them as waves of breath that cause your belly to soften and inflate, your ribcage to extend up and out to the sides, and your upper chest and throat to expand slightly. Soon you will notice that your breath flows naturally in this pattern and you may find yourself breathing this way even when you are not engaging in your practice of the Five Tibetans.

Restoration and Transformation

While the "rest poses" are places to bring your breath and heart rate back to a normal rhythm, they will also, most likely, create opportunities for transformation. My personal experience has been that deeply embedded and rich emotions tend to bubble up when I am in Child's Pose or Corpse Pose. What causes those emotions to surface?

In Chapter 2 you will review information about the chakras associated with the Five Tibetans. The chakras are energy centers in the body that can become clogged by held hurts and painful emotions. As you mindfully address each chakra and perform the Five Tibetans, emotions that have been "stuck" may shift. The rest poses provide a perfect setting for letting those emotions flow and go. It is not uncommon to feel tears surfacing or anger erupting as you move into a rest pose. That is a perfect time to invoke visualizations or meditations that will support your clearing or transforming of those feelings. To aid that transformation, I will provide a visualization that you can do while you are in the rest pose after each of the Five Tibetans. You may want to experiment with doing and not doing the visualizations to see what works best for you. I suggest you keep notes in your journey journal about your experiences in the rest poses.

The First Tibetan

The First Tibetan has a different character from the four that follow. It seems more like child's play than a yoga pose. If you have ever seen the Whirling Dervishes of Sufi culture, you have a basic idea of the First Tibetan. In essence, the First Tibetan is a series of clockwise spins.

To begin the First Tibetan, you will stand up straight with your arms extended from your sides and parallel to the floor. Your palms will be facing down. You will move around in a clockwise direction, either pivoting on the balls of your feet or holding one heel in place. You will start with three spins and explore what works for you. Go slowly at first. You can build up speed as your tolerance increases. Rest in Child's Pose after you have completed your spins.

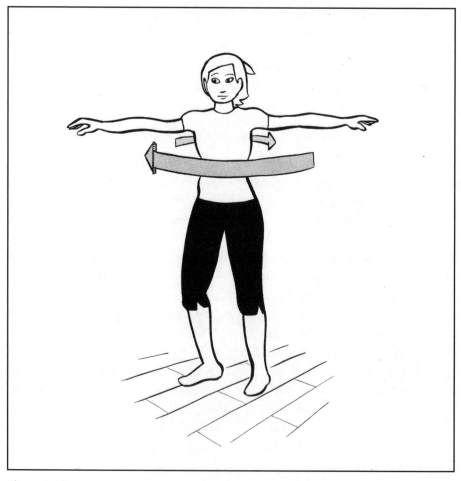

The First Tibetan

Breathing in the First Tibetan is apparently based on personal preference. Some teachers suggest holding your breath as you do the spins; others, me included, breathe with the spins. If I slow my process down and look at it more carefully, I realize I tend to inhale for two spins and exhale on the next two spins. The key to sticking with the Five Tibetans as a practice is in finding what works for you. Take time to experiment with how you feel in the spins and where the breathing seems most effective.

When you begin performing the First Tibetan, you may need to explore ways to reduce dizziness and nausea. The classic solution is to incorporate the technique used by dancers and skaters, i.e., to focus your eyes on a point in front of you and then snap your head around at the end. Another strategy is to keep your eyes on the hand that is leading the spin. What has worked best for me is to sight a point out in front of me in the beginning, go into the spin, and then let my eyes reconnect with the focal point each time I come back around to the starting point. I encourage you to remain curious and discover the way that best suits you. If you are feeling dizzy after the spins, you can relieve the discomfort by placing your hands on your hips and breathing out hard as you bend forward. Two or three forceful exhalations will reduce the dizziness and nausea.

If you find that you cannot do the spins without feeling excessively dizzy, begin by standing in place and swaying your arms back and forth as you turn from side to side. As you build experience and confidence with the other poses, you can try the First Tibetan again. While the Five Tibetans are separate poses, they are also impacting your body as a whole. With regular practice of the poses that you can do, you will find it easier to add in the poses that seemed difficult when you first set out.

The Second Tibetan

Those of you who will read or have read Peter Kelder's book will note that he refers to the Second Tibetan as the "Fourth Rite." The reason for this will be more apparent as we progress in the workshop, but I have reordered the sequence of the yogas to better address the Western mindset and to create a smooth flow through the chakras. This will not matter if you have not read other books on the Five Tibetans, but is a heads up for those of you with prior experience.

The Second Tibetan is similar to Reverse Table Pose in Hatha yoga. This is a pose that many people find particularly difficult. If it doesn't come at first, play with alternatives and continue to practice the other poses. In time, you will find that you are able to perform the pose with greater ease.

You begin the Second Tibetan sitting upright on the mat, with your legs stretched out in front of you and your hands at your sides, palms on the floor. As you inhale, bring your hips up while keeping your feet flat on the mat. Your head should go back as far as is comfortable, but you should not overextend the neck. Once in the pose, your head, torso, and thighs will create a tablelike surface. You will exhale as you move your hips back down and assume your original sitting position. Rest in Corpse Pose after you complete your repetitions of the Second Tibetan.

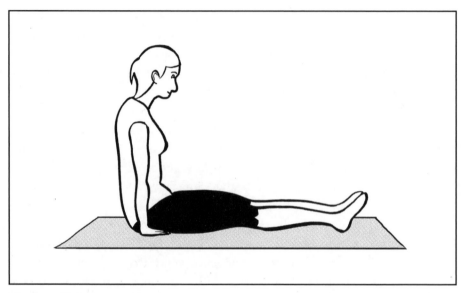

The Second Tibetan – step 1

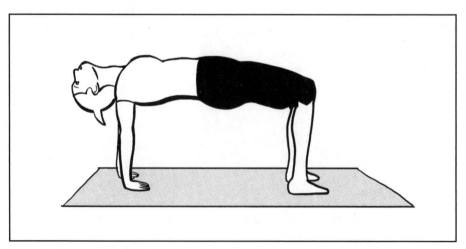

The Second Tibetan – step 2

The Second Tibetan will help you build core strength and stamina. It may take a few weeks to get there. If you have injuries to your shoulders or back, be very careful as you proceed. If you feel any pain or discomfort in your wrists, shift your hand position. Try angling your hands away from your body and involving your fingers more in the lift. Spread your fingers and press into your finger pads and the mounds at the base of your fingers (knuckle pads). This action of engaging your fingers will protect your wrists. There are also several alternative body postures for this pose. If you are able to make it up into the "table" part, but it seems awkward or strenuous, place a yoga block or rolled towel under your hands. It might be that you need more arm length. If getting your hips off the mat seems impossible, move your feet in two or three inches toward your hips, lift your hips off the mat, and then swing back down to sitting. If even that seems too much, push your chest out and up as you inhale and move your chest back down as you exhale. Only do what is comfortable for you. Only extend yourself as far as seems physically and emotionally safe.

When I first began doing this pose, I did not understand why some people found it so difficult. I arose into it easily. While I was writing this book, however, I experienced a shoulder injury. The pain of doing the Second Tibetan brought tears to my eyes when I lay down in the rest pose afterwards. I found myself dreading the pose. I also discovered that my discomfort with this pose influenced my enthusiasm for the other poses. In time, my shoulder healed and I was once again able to fully engage in the practice. It was a good lesson on many levels. If you have shoulder injuries, I encourage you to keep working with this pose. Find a way to keep it safely in your repertoire. As we will see in Chapter 2, the shoulders are linked to the heart chakra. It is possible, then, that a sore shoulder is speaking to you about an issue of the heart.

The Third Tibetan

A teacher once referred to the Third Tibetan as a "chiropractor's dream." While that might tend to scare you away, what I want to do is encourage you to be attentive and mindful as you perform this pose. The Third Tibetan is somewhat similar to Camel Pose in Hatha yoga. It is the pose that appears on the cover of Christopher Kilham's book, *The Five Tibetans,* and likely the one that creates angst in the mind of the beholder. I will teach you the Third Tibetan as I was taught to do the pose. You will find another rendition of this pose in Kelder's book.

You will begin the Third Tibetan from a kneeling position on your mat. You may choose to lay the tops of your feet on the mat or tuck your toes under, so that your feet are up off the surface. The starting position for the pose is to hold an erect spine and to rest your chin on your chest. Place your hands on your hips, with your thumbs resting lightly on the two divots on either side of the spine. (You will form "wings" with your arms, as my friend and dedicated Five Tibetan Workshop participant Maggie says.) By positioning your hands on your back in this way, you have created additional support for your lower back.

You will start the pose by inhaling and letting your elbows guide you backward. Please note that this means you will be leading with your arms and not with your head. As your arms go back, your chest will open and your heart will move upward. You will only extend back as far as is comfortable. (Do not go all the way back, as you would in Camel Pose.) Keep your thighs as straight (vertically) as possible as you arch your back.

When you are ready, you will exhale as you carefully come back up into the starting position. Again, lead with your "wings," and not with your neck. Bring your heart forward, not your head, so there is no snapping the neck back into place. The restorative pose for Third Tibetan is Child's Pose.

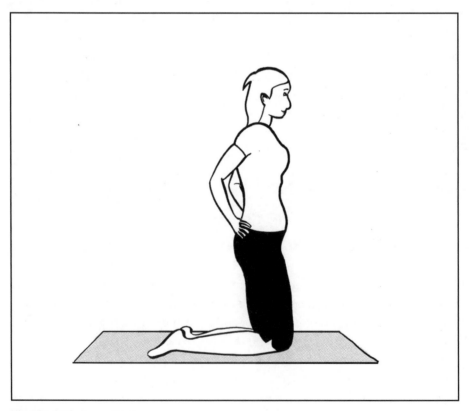

The Third Tibetan – step 1

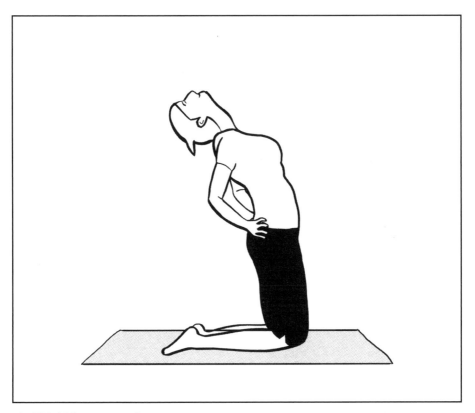

The Third Tibetan – step 2

If you have lower back problems, carefully explore this pose, noticing any strain or discomfort that might arise. Keeping your thighs perpendicular to the floor will take strain off the lower back as you return to the starting position. Protect the lower back by lengthening through the spine, particularly the lower back, and not crunching or narrowing the space there. If you are uncomfortable with the pose in the beginning, start by pushing your chest out and up on the inhale and then returning to the start position.

The Fourth Tibetan

Several of my clients find the Fourth Tibetan to be their favorite. Don't let that fool you! You will build core strength doing this pose. To begin the Fourth Tibetan, lie flat on your back on your mat with your legs stretched out, feet together, arms along your sides, and palms flat on the floor. On the inhalation, raise your head and torso and then raise your legs straight up into the air. Keep your legs straight and flex your feet by pointing your heels at the ceiling. You can extend the pose beyond 90 degrees, if that is comfortable for you. When you are ready to unfold, you will exhale and bring your head and feet back to the mat at the same time. Move into Corpse Pose to rest.

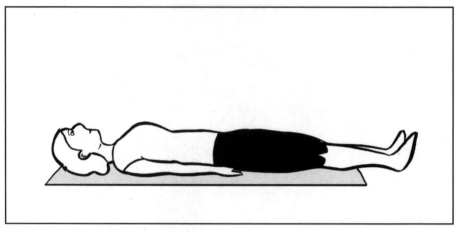

The Fourth Tibetan – step 1

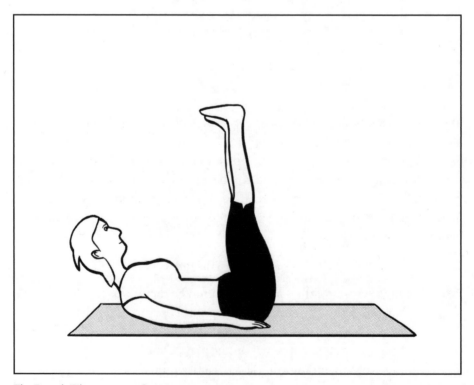

The Fourth Tibetan – step 2

I make a modification to this pose when I do it in my practice. I place my hands (palms down) under the top of my hips to provide more support. You could also add a pillow or a blanket roll. I use this variation when I teach the Five Tibetans to decrease the likelihood of an injury or strain to the lower back.

Fifth Tibetan

If I have a favorite Tibetan, it is the Fifth. This pose is a blend of two Hatha yoga poses: Upward-Facing Dog and Downward-Facing Dog. The Fifth Tibetan strengthens the arms, wrists, and back. Horsley contends that it reduces fat in the abdominals as well. (I am still waiting for that to happen.) The Fifth Tibetan is a rigorous, but pleasurable, end to the sequence.

I begin the Fifth Tibetan on my hands and knees. I say "I begin" because other teachers may have you begin on your stomach and push up into the Upward-Facing Dog Pose to start or initiate the pose. Beginning on my hands and knees puts me in position for the mantra for the Fifth Tibetan. From the hands-and-knees start, stretch out your legs behind you and place your feet hip distance apart, toes tucked. Let your body relax and sag in between your arms, and let your head and back arch backward (to a comfortable place).

In the beginning you may wish to let your thighs and knees rest on the mat. When you are feeling stronger, you can hold your legs off the mat. From the "sag," you will inhale and use your shoulders and upper back to help you lift your buttocks into the air and stand up on your toes.

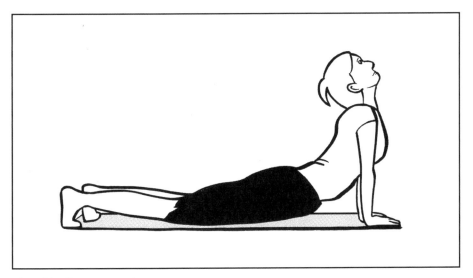

The Fifth Tibetan – step 1

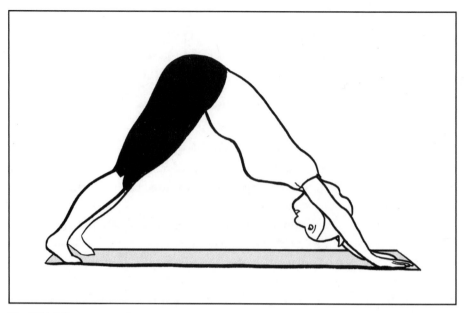

The Fifth Tibetan – step 2

Your hands and feet will remain in their starting place. As you move into the pose you will fold your head inward between your arms until your chin is tucked on your chest. You will resemble an inverted V at this point. When you are ready to unfold, you will exhale and return to the start position, allowing your head and back to arch slightly. Recover by moving into Child's Pose.

There are varying perspectives on whether your heels should be down (as in a traditional Downward-Facing Dog Pose) or up. The original drawings in Kelder's books show the heels down. In *Chakra Workout*, Mary Horsley specifies that the heels should be up. Try both ways and determine which has the greatest impact on you. I began by using Kelder's rendition and now integrate Horsley's modeling of the pose in my practice. I can feel the difference in the extension of the buttocks and hamstrings.

Creating Your Practice

There is no right way to begin practicing the Five Tibetans. I suggest a 12-week scenario in order to parallel the contents of this book, but the best practice is the one that works for you. Keep in mind that there are two reasons for creating your daily practice: to benefit physically from the daily execution of the poses and to transform your thinking through contemplation of the mantras. Each of those activities is an essential part of the process.

WEEK 1

One of the most important preliminary activities for developing any practice is the creation of a time and a space in which to do your work. You will need at least 30 minutes a day to start with, and you may find that you will want more time as you progress. You will need privacy (even if you are working with a partner) and a yoga mat or towel. Consider burning candles and incense and playing your favorite meditative music. Spend time visualizing your perfect space and ambience. You will also need to determine a time for your practice. For me, the early morning is best. However, we all have different schedules and responsibilities. Perhaps your best time is right after the children go to school or while the baby naps. In the workplace, you could consider closing your office door and doing the Five Tibetans during the lunch hour. Many people perform the Five Tibetans before going to bed. The only essential element of your time selection is that you can adhere to it most of the time.

Once you have created your space and have determined the best time, commit yourself to going in at the appointed time each day of Week 1 in order to create a habit. During that time, you can try out the poses and find the positions that work best for you. If you are using this book as the basis for your own workshop, I suggest you also read Chapters 1 and 2, and watch the introductory video on the website (*www.5tibetansworkshop.com*).

WEEK 2

With a week of logistics and habit-making behind you, you are ready to put it all together to establish your personal practice. In Week 2, perform three repetitions of each of the Five Tibetans, if possible. Include the rest poses after each of the Tibetans. Pay attention to your breathing and the rhythm of your breath as you repeat each pose. Practice saying the mantras I have provided in Chapter 2 before each of the poses. You may want to write the mantras out on paper or note cards. Read Chapter 3 to develop an understanding of the grasping and healing behaviors.

WEEKS 3 – 12

Once you have a routine in place, you can focus on increasing the number of repetitions of each Tibetan and saying the accompanying mantras. When I began doing the Five Tibetans, I followed the directions in Kelder's book, i.e., I began with three repetitions of each pose and increased the number of repetitions by two each week. If you follow that prescription, you will theoretically be doing 21 repetitions of the Five Tibetans at the end of week 12.

Remember to be patient and gentle with yourself. Regardless of the number of repetitions of the Five Tibetans you can do, you are establishing a practice. If you choose to align reading this book with increasing the number of repetitions, read Chapter 4 in Week 3 and then read one chapter each week thereafter. As you progress through the book and practice the Five Tibetans, you can consciously make the content of each chapter part of your contemplations both on and off your yoga mat each week.

CHAPTER 2

The Chakras and Transformational Elements

According to Peter Kelder's mentor, Colonel Bradford, the goal of performing the Five Rites (our Five Tibetans) was to balance and increase the rotations of the seven spinning energy vortexes that we know as "chakras" (*chakra* is the Sanskrit word for "wheel"). Spinning 3–4 inches outside the body, the chakras are directly connected to the nervous system and govern the ductless endocrine glands.

When we are young, the chakras are clear and bright and spin at great speeds, but they dull and slow as we age. In *Shaman, Healer, Sage*, Alberto Villoldo explains that as we endure the losses and disappointments of life, "toxic residue" is left behind. The resulting "sludge" attaches to the chakras and impedes their vibration or speed of rotation. It reminds me of the old drain cleaner ad for removing greasy buildup, except here the energy pipes get clogged and the flow of vital energy, or *prana*, is restricted. According to the colonel, his five exercises increased the velocity of the chakras and, thereby, created health and vitality.

While I will venture that most people reading this book are familiar with the concept of chakras, I want to address the topic here to provide information that relates directly to the Five Tibetans and to the mantras that you will be learning in the following chapters. There are numerous references on the subject of the chakras. For this chapter, I identified a range of perspectives and arranged them into a framework that best describes what I consider to be the work of each of the Five Tibetans. I have only provided you with a fraction of the information about this intriguing and complex subject. Should you be interested, you will find resources in the bibliography that will point you to additional information.

While most of us are familiar with the seven main chakras that Colonel Bradford referred to, different spiritual traditions recognize more or fewer chakras in the body. In Tibetan Buddhism, varying practices include as few as four and as many as 10 chakras. Here, we will work with the five chakras that correspond to the poses of the Five Tibetans.

Traditionally, discussions of the chakras begin with the root, or first, chakra and proceed upward. Hatha yoga practice is meant to move the Kundalini energy in the root chakra upward to the crown chakra. Your practice with the Five Tibetans, however, will begin with contemplations of the Third Eye and move downward to the root chakra. As I researched an explanation for this reversal, I learned that in some Tibetan traditions, the physical practice is intentionally designed to bring energy down from the crown into the lower chakras.

Although they are five distinct exercises, the Five Tibetans work together as a whole. Likewise, the chakras reviewed here also work together as a whole. In Colonel Bradford's account, the First Tibetan, the spin, serves to align all the chakras. His description did not pair each rite with a specific chakra; I have added that approach according to the system taught by Dekyi-Lee Oldershaw. Identifying each of the Five Tibetans with a specific chakra encourages attention to the contemplative work of the yoga.

The use of sacred elements (light, air, fire, water, and earth) to accompany the Five Tibetans and the chakras is consistent with Tibetan practice. Using the elements in your own daily practice allows you to integrate their sacred essence into the transformational work of looking deeply into and committing to a life of nonattachment, nonresistance, and nonpermanence. I will briefly describe the elements associated with each of the Five Tibetans and their chakra focus. The connections of the elements, the chakras, and the yoga poses will be expanded further as we explore the individual grasping and healing behaviors in Chapters 4–13.

The First Tibetan –
Third Eye and Pure Light

The First Tibetan is paired with the sixth chakra, known as the Third Eye. Located between and slightly above the brow, and projecting out from the pituitary and pineal glands, the Third Eye is considered the seat of enlightenment and insight. The Sanskrit word for the Third Eye is *ajna,* meaning "unlimited power." This chakra is associated with the color indigo. Purple and deep blue gemstones, such as amethyst, sapphire, and lapis lazuli, are connected to the Third Eye. Applying aromatherapy oils such as hyacinth, violet, rosemary, and mint, and eating red-purple foods (e.g., blueberries, grapes, and blackcurrants) will help balance this chakra.

People with active sixth chakras are resolute, decisive, and undivided in their thinking and actions. They live in a state of nonduality and understand that everything is interconnected and as it is meant to be. Intuition is a guiding force. Clair-voyance (intuitive insights), clairaudience (intuitive hearing), and clairsentience (intuitive feeling) are often well developed.

The Third Eye is perhaps the most mystical of the major chakras, as it is considered to be a portal into your awareness and knowing of yourself and the spiritual realms. Through it, you realize the divine presence within you and experience the Divine in others. You are able to perceive the events happening around you as merely experiences, thereby able to remain curious without succumbing to drama and confusion. The stories of the mind have less hold on you. You can act with loving detachment, no longer propelled by doubt, fear, grasping, and aversion.

While the positive attributes of an active Third Eye are impressive, the negative expressions can be quite debilitating. An overactive Third Eye may result in self-aggrandizement, headaches, depression, delusions, obsessions, and "analysis paralysis." Nightmares may persist in the dream life. Memory and cognition may be impacted. A person with an underfunctioning Third Eye chakra may be carried away by the stories of the moment, unable to reel in the mind and manage fears or reactions to the events happening around her.

Pure light is the transformational element associated with the First Tibetan. Light is technically not one of the earth elements, but it is frequently used to represent the power and scope of the Third Eye. Light brings us out of the darkness and illuminates the aspects of self and others that might otherwise escape our notice. In drawings, insight is often represented by light or a light bulb over the head. We recognize that light enhances our vision and heightens our awareness. In your work with the First Tibetan, you will call on the light element to open the Third Eye, illuminate confusion, and light the way for insight.

The Second Tibetan – Heart Chakra and the Air Element

The heart chakra is located in the middle of the chest (not over the physical heart) and the center of the chakra plane. Above the heart chakra are chakras that govern our connections to spirit and our higher selves (throat, Third Eye, and crown). Below the heart chakra are the chakras that create our sense of security in the physical world and in our relationship with our families and others (solar plexus, sacral, and root).

An open and active heart chakra allows movement of energy both up from the root chakra and down from the crown chakra. A blocked heart chakra creates a constriction in the flow of energy from above and below, creating all manner of emotional and physical problems, including depression, lack of forgiveness and compassion, resentment, abuse, asthma, heart disease, and immune deficiencies. As you will see in Chapter 10, a closed heart chakra also impacts the way you see yourself and the degree to which you can allow yourself the gift of vulnerability. An under-functioning heart chakra can lead to your inability to believe in your own worth and be with your own imperfections.

You need only look around you to see our society's preoccupation with all things of the heart. This symbol for love is ubiquitous; we find it everywhere and on just about everything. The word "love" is used to describe a range of emotions from how we feel about the chocolate we are eating to the way we experience our partners and families. The love expressed by an open heart chakra, however, is not that kind of love. It is more akin to the "loving detachment" of the Third Eye chakra. Persons with open heart chakras are compassionate and forgiving, but neither grasping nor attaching. They are able to both give and receive love freely.

The heart chakra is governed by the thymus gland. As this gland is involved in cell-mediated immunity, there is a correlation between the functioning of the heart chakra and physical wellness. You may notice the saying "Open your heart, heal your life" in my promotional materials. The heart chakra is the metaphorical gateway to creating healthier relationships and a healthier you. This chakra is also associated with the lungs and the limbs and body parts that are attached to your central cardiothoracic core, including the shoulders, breasts, arms, wrists, and hands. It is easy to see why an imbalanced heart chakra can have a significant impact on your health and daily functioning.

The Sanskrit word for the heart chakra is *anahata,* meaning "unstruck" or "unbeaten" or "unbound." A healthy heart chakra allows us to let go of material things and bask in the presence of joy and love and peace. This chakra is associated with the color green (as well as pink). Rose quartz, emerald, jade, and malachite gemstones help activate the heart chakra as do aromatics, such as rosewater, bergamot, clary sage, and geranium. Foods that support the heart chakra include green cruciferous and leafy vegetables, avocados, sprouts, beans, and grains. A heart-healthy diet will enhance the activity of your heart chakra.

The heart chakra is referred to as the "gateway of the winds"; air is its representative element. Sit back for a moment and close your eyes. Think about air. What does it feel like? Smell like? Sound like? Taste like? While it is hard to describe, we know our lives depend on it. Physiologically, we can live without food and water for a time; we cannot live without air for more than a few minutes.

On a different level, as a former physics teacher, I can say with confidence that air has weight and takes up space. Hence, it is considered to be matter. This usually invisible material that surrounds us every minute of the day may not seem like much, but air can pack quite a punch. In fact, the pressure of the air around you right now is exerting a constant force on your body equivalent to 14.7 pounds per square inch. I guess you could say air matters and *is* matter. It matters to your health and to your heart.

This element creates a beautiful picture of what is required to open the heart chakra. We will work more with this metaphor later in Chapters 5 and 12, but suffice it to say that air transforms the space and place it is in. For example, visualize taking the complete breath that you learned in Chapter 1. Consider how the air you draw into your body is impacting your own form. Your belly swells. Your chest expands. As you exhale, the air takes with it stale carbon dioxide and water vapor. As the representative element of the heart chakra, air creates a natural picture of expansion and cleansing.

Beyond creating more space and clearing away undesirable remains, the air element brings forth transformation. The familiar expression "winds of change" underscores the notion that air carries revolution. According to the Bön tradition in Tibetan Buddhism, when the air element is balanced you are more likely to shift anger, depression, and self-pity into more positive thoughts and emotions. Your anxiety or worry can move effortlessly on to resolution and flexibility; you know the next thing is already on its way. There is no "stuckness." You are free to move in new directions and take on varying perspectives.

Your daily practice of the Second Tibetan will allow you to explore your relationship with the air element. Your inhalations will expand your chest as you move up into the pose. I will encourage you as we work with this pose to notice your breathing. Is it tight? Constricted? Does your chest feel expansive? Is your air heavy or do you find that the breath easily enters you? The close alliance between the air element and the heart chakra provides you with opportunities to connect with your breath and to explore the way your emotions are either constricting or allowing the flow of air into your body and being.

The Third Tibetan – Solar Plexus Chakra and The Fire Element

The solar plexus, or *manipura* in Saskrit, is located in the area beneath the ribs and just above the navel. It is the powerhouse of chakras in terms of the organs that are associated with it. Its primary organ is the pancreas, the gland responsible for producing insulin, the hormone that helps cells metabolize glucose into energy. However, this chakra also resides in the realm of the stomach, liver, gall bladder, and spleen. It rules digestion, the storing and releasing of food energy, and the purification of the body's liquid stores. You can see quite quickly why imbalances in the third chakra manifest as a range of physical ailments, including gastrointestinal irregularities, eating disorders, blood diseases, diabetes, liver problems, and gall stones. This chakra is, quite literally, the center of our existence.

The solar plexus chakra did not exist in the Five Tibetans program as I learned it—in the original system, the Third Tibetan, as I have described it here, was actually paired with the fifth chakra, the throat chakra (a chakra that I am not covering here). After a discussion with my editor, Sabine Weeke, we decided that the Third Tibetan actually is more closely connected to the traditional third chakra (solar plexus chakra) of the Hindu system. One explanation for this seeming disparity is that in Eastern spirituality, there is no pressing need to work with the solar plexus chakra; in Western culture, however, this is where most of us live—struggling with and exploring our personal power.

When the third chakra is balanced, you are able to manifest your own destiny. You have a sense that you can accomplish anything you set your mind to, and you do. There is a warrior archetype attached to this chakra. You are fearless. You battle. You achieve. You are sure of yourself.

The negative expressions are relatively obvious. When the energy in the third chakra is excessive, an overexpression of confidence and personal power can result. We may notice an inflated ego; domineering, dictatorial, or tyrannical behavior; or pursuits for the sake of power and fame. Exaggerated assertiveness or aggressiveness may emerge. Such articulation of this chakra can perhaps be best characterized by "power over"—our hidden bully lurks nearby. If, on the other hand, our third chakra is underfunctioning, we may feel alone, scared, full of shame and guilt, insecure, dependent, and easily discouraged. Either way, a lack of balance in the solar plexus chakra will have a marked impact on our achievements and our relationships.

I want to mention at this point that each of us will probably be able to identify with both the over- and underfunctioning aspects of the third chakra. It is happening to me as I write this. I can pinpoint situations where I am aggressive, when I fail to use my compassionate voice and I overstep my personal power. At other times I retreat in shyness and insecurity. Once in a while I feel balanced, manage my ego, and move mountains without taking any casualties. I am going to assert that this is normal. (It makes me feel better.) So when you read through the list, please notice what is relevant for you and then move on. As we go along in the workshop, you may want to revisit this section of the book and take your observations into your daily practice.

The color associated with the third chakra is yellow (and gold). Yellow gemstones such as amber, tiger-eye, agate, and topaz, as well as natural oils like bergamot, lemon, chamomile, and thyme are helpful for balancing the energy of the solar plexus chakra. Eating yellow foods (corn, yellow peppers, summer squash, and citrus) supports this chakra. Sour foods, legumes, and whole grains also help keep the third chakra open and functioning at a high level. It is important to note here that sugary and processed foods, starchy carbohydrates, and caffeine can take away from the effectiveness of the energy storing and burning aspects of the pancreas. As a result, these foods can render us tired or overagitated, unable to step into or step back from our expression of personal power. If you are sensing that your solar plexus chakra is out of balance, you may wish to first examine your daily diet.

Fire is the element that coincides with the solar plexus chakra. Using the expression "she has a fire in her belly" to describe someone who is going after a goal tells us that the person is moving forward with conviction and a sense that nothing can detour her from her course. She is eager, ambitious, and confident. When the inner fires of the third chakra are burning, we are able to create and initiate. We are enthusiastic and excited by our own existence—blissful in our bodies and joyful of the opportunities in each new day. We can, however, experience either a surplus or a lack of fire. Too much fire can render us irritable or agitated. We will have a tendency to lash out or react in anger. We cannot relax or sit in silence. When fire is deficient, we may experience a lack of enjoyment, a paucity of new ideas and inspirations, and a lack of enthusiasm about life in general.

Fourth Tibetan –
Sacral Chakra and the Water Element

The sacral chakra (*svadisthana*) is located four fingers below the navel and is associated with the sexual and lower digestive organs, the kidneys, and the lower back. The testes and ovaries are the glands that govern this second chakra. From this fertile energy womb we bring forth creativity, sexuality, and pleasure. When it is in balance, we are joyful, resilient, playful, appropriately sensual, and flexible. When the second chakra is underfunctioning or overfunctioning, we can experience sexual problems, fear, uncertainty, lack of trust, persistent back pain, bladder and urinary issues, and a general sense of worthlessness.

The sacral chakra vibrates to a rich orange color and is nurtured and balanced by succulent orange-red foods (e.g., salmon, carrots, yams, oranges, and pomegranates). Eating seeds, tropical fruits, and nuts also has a therapeutic effect on this chakra. Fragrant oils such as sandalwood, jasmine, and rose aid in releasing the creative and sensual energy residing in the second chakra.

Issues related to money and integrity manifest in the sacral chakra. When this chakra is unbalanced, we can confuse personal value with financial assets and may be willing to compromise ourselves (or others) for the sake of money. In her book *Sacred Contracts*, Caroline Myss asserts that we all possess a universal archetype called the "Prostitute." As its name suggests, the Prostitute archetype is about selling yourself—or selling yourself out—to gain financial security or control of others. Staying in an abusive relationship or continuing in a job where you are asked to be unethical solely for the purpose of financial security would be examples of the Prostitute in action. From a stronger place in a balanced sacral chakra, however, the Prostitute represents our commitment to ourselves and our integrity. We learn that we can say "No" and that our love and our talents are not for sale. We can stand in our unwavering belief that we have innate value and can live in alignment with our true selves. The fact that the Sanskrit word *svadisthana* means "dwelling place of the self" indicates that our highest and best selves are at home in the sacral chakra.

The sacral chakra is matched with the water element. Unlike the other elements, water is literally within us. Our bodies and our planet are primarily made of water. It is our place of origin; we developed in the water of our mother's womb. Water flows from place to place, cleanses us when we are dirty, and refreshes us when we are tired and thirsty. Similarly, when the water element is balanced, we can "go with the flow" and be accepting of our circumstances. We move easily in and out of life's transitions without losing our joy and contentment. We tend to enjoy life and all of its dimensions. We are comfortable with ourselves and the people around us. Too much water can leave us weepy and emotional, caught up in transient emotions. When water is in excess, we might also experience a sense of exaggerated contentment leading to a lack of productivity. A deficiency of water results in a "dry" life experience. We are not comfortable with ourselves, our lives, or the people around us. Our "well of life" needs to be filled with sweetness, creativity, and joy.

The Fifth Tibetan –
Root Chakra and The Earth Element

The Fifth Tibetan is associated with what is traditionally considered the first, or root, chakra and is governed by the adrenal glands. Home of the Kundalini energy, the root chakra is located in the base of the spine. The roots of the first chakra extend downward, deep into the solid layers of Mother Earth who provides a picture of the essence of this energy center, i.e., this is the place where our early experiences with nurturing and sense of kinship are recorded.

The root chakra oversees the lower intestines and the solid body parts, including the spine and bones. The feet and legs are important instruments of the root chakra; your survival once depended on your ability to flee danger. The root chakra represents your most primal, instinctual self and regulates your most basic needs: food, shelter, and survival. Your sense of the world as a safe place and your ability to connect to the people around you starts here.

The Sanskrit word for the root chakra is *muladhara*, or "foundation." When the root chakra is balanced, we know that we are secure and loved and that our needs will be taken care of. We enjoy a sense of connection to the earth and to the people around us and express gratitude for the bounty that surrounds us. When this chakra is not in balance, we may be prone to insecurity and fear. Scarcity or materialism may result from a feeling that we can never have enough. The blocked energy of the root chakra can lead to disorders of the bowels, the bones, and the circulation.

The root chakra vibrates a bright red. Wearing red clothing is one way you can bring the energy of the first chakra into your awareness. Eating root vegetables and foods with a deep red color will assist the balance of the root chakra as will holding or wearing red gemstones, such as agate, garnet, ruby, and bloodstone. Dabbing on "earthy" oils (e.g., musk, patchouli, myrrh, and lavender) can also elevate the energy of this chakra. An activity as simple as walking barefoot in the grass will help you create a stronger sense of your connection to the earth and will enhance the energy of the root chakra.

It should not be surprising that the root chakra is associated with the earth element. Our sense of "being grounded" gives us a picture of possessing sufficient earth element. We are centered, stable, and balanced. We exhibit a spirit of equanimity. Our confidence and knowledge are not easily shaken. We are responsible to ourselves and others and are not given to impulsiveness. When there is too much earth we may be too "heavy," unable to move or think, and prone to getting "stuck" in daily practices or relationships because change is overwhelming. Too little earth results in being "airy-fairy" and flighty. We are not able to complete our tasks, or we have a general sense of dissatisfaction. In such cases, there may be a need to seek stability in solid relationships or communities.

The Practice Scaffold

Familiarizing yourself with the poses of the Five Tibetans, the chakras, and the transformational elements is an essential first step before you begin the daily practice of contemplating the behaviors outlined in this book. You might think of the Five Tibetans as a physical scaffold that supports you as you exercise and invigorate your chakras. Daily practice of the Five Tibetans provides a time, place, and space to contemplate the dissolution and transformation of behaviors that are not serving your relationships or your life. During that time you will also become more mindful of the positive behaviors able to move you away from past hurtful and destructive patterns and into a life of greater joy and connection. Let's now explore the grasping and healing behaviors that form the core of the purpose of your practice in the Five Tibetan Yogas Workshop.

CHAPTER 3

Grasping and Healing

I am easily seduced by a nicely starched, button-up white shirt. There is some-thing so lovely and alluring about it. Maybe it is the whiteness. Or the hint of stiffness. Regardless, I am more likely to let go of a sizeable sum of money for one of these than any other piece of clothing. I currently have such a shirt. I wore it to a family Easter luncheon. When I got home, I noticed a spot between the second and third buttons.

I was disappointed by it. It was my favorite shirt. Now, its whiteness had been impaired by this spot of unknown origin or composition. I tried to get it out. I used all the homemade, environmentally friendly remedies I could think of and washed it two or three times. But each time I pulled it out of the washer, the spot was still there.

I was on the move at the time, so I folded the shirt with its spot and put it in my suitcase. When I opened the suitcase to get out something to wear, I no-ticed the shirt, thought about the spot, then opted for something else. The shirt remained as it was for a couple of months. Every time I considered wearing it, I was aware of thinking that I would not be comfortable in it. People would notice its blemish. I would know the spot was there. I would be self-conscious. Its pure whiteness had been sullied. While it really was a fairly light stain, in my mind it ruined the shirt.

As I prepared materials for our workshops and for this book, I pondered the best way to describe "grasping" behaviors. It's essential to be able to create a clear picture of what these behaviors represent, because they are the real work of this book. The easiest explanation is that grasping behaviors are derivations of the Buddhist concept of "delusion." According to the Dalai Lama, delusions "are states of mind which … leave us disturbed, confused, or unhappy." My Western sense-making mind has determined that delusions result from our need to control our environment or the outcome of our circumstances. They are us grasping at or trying to hold onto people or things or ideas. They impair our functioning in the world and our happiness by ultimately cutting us off from the love and compassion and connection we have been created to experience and share. How, exactly, do they do all that damage?

As I opened my suitcase time after time and did not choose the white shirt, I began to understand how the grasping behaviors steal our joy. There it was—my beautiful white shirt. I looked good in that shirt. I felt attractive in the shirt. But once I became self-conscious about the spot, I put the shirt away in the suitcase and kept it locked up, unused.

In Part II of this book, you will explore the five grasping behaviors that represent the down-and-dirty work of each of the Five Tibetans: *confusion, resentment, doubt, fear,* and *miserliness.* I am going to propose that in each case, there is a spot. A stain. A past hurt or slight or devastation. Perhaps a time that you had needs that were not met. Maybe a person who was meant to keep you safe and who, instead, brought physical or emotional pain. The spots can be tiny or large, but they all have the same result: they cause you to put away the best parts of yourself, wear other colors and shy away from your true feelings and self. Each of the grasping behaviors has the potential to not only steal your joy, but steal your life as well.

Finally, I took the shirt out of the suitcase, determined to eradicate that spot. I again tried all the home-spun remedies. I am sure some of you are telling me what to do right now. In the end, I had to go right at it with a Q-tip soaked in bleach, my mother's suggestion. I had been afraid to do that in the beginning, as bleach can sometimes cause a spot to darken rather than remove it. But, in this case, the spot disappeared. The shirt was washed one more time and once again hangs out in the open ready to be worn and enjoyed.

Ignoring our spots, pretending they are not there, and putting away the parts of ourselves we do not feel comfortable displaying, all lead to rifts in our authenticity and our sense that the world is a safe place. I encourage you to go courageously into the work of the grasping behaviors. In the case of my shirt, I finally had to apply strong and direct attention right on the spot. I literally painted the bleach just within the boundaries of that stain. Similarly, you will have an opportunity in this book to focus your attention directly on some of the peskiest, most destructive behaviors in the human realm. The only approach I know for addressing them is to liberally apply the "bleach" of mindfulness to each one, to give it its due, to not shrink back from utilizing the strongest cleanser available: *love.* In each case, I will encourage you to remember Thich Nhat Hanh's instruction to cradle your hurts and your own behaviors as you would a precious newborn. They are part of who you are. They are here as your teachers.

The two grasping behaviors that I think are especially resistant to "treatment" are resentment and miserliness. These behaviors do not usually make the top 10 self-help lists. In my conversations with people about the grasping behaviors, these are the two least-claimed activities. We know being angry is okay, but holding resentment feels a little less "nice." What kinds of people hold resentment? All kinds of people. All people. It is a natural artifact of our inner child's need for self-protection. Each one of us will have a resentment spot or two to deal with.

What about the grasping behavior of miserliness? Where does miserliness show up in my life? When I think of miserliness I imagine old man Scrooge in his nightgown shivering in the snow of Christmas Future. At first, I was going to pair isolation with the Fifth Tibetan. But the more I pondered the main players of disconnection in my own life, the more miserliness came to the forefront. Resentment and miserliness are close companions. Withholding ourselves, our love, our money, our compassion, our forgiveness. A little here and a little there; sooner or later it will create noticeable tension in our lives and relationships. So, go boldly. It is a Star Trek experience—few people will have been there before you.

On the heels of your work with the grasping behaviors will come their antidotes, the healing behaviors. If you are thinking that the hard part will be behind you, be prepared for a shock when you begin looking at *awareness, vulnerability, surrender, authenticity,* and *connection.* Now there's some *wuk* to do! Each of these behaviors will be linked to the characteristics of the chakras that represent the Five Tibetans' poses. Your focus will be to dissolve and transform the behaviors you want to put to rest into thoughts and actions that will serve you. As you do the Five Tibetans each day, you will be contemplating the way your Third Eye, heart, solar plexus, sacral, and root chakras are opening in response to your intentions for healing and growth.

My top two star healing behaviors are surrender and authenticity. Being with what is and being who you were created to be require consistent spiritual focus and clearing. Surrender forces us to explore nonpermanence in all its pleasant and not-so-pleasant forms. The road to authenticity goes straight through nonattachment. We have to let go of what other people think about us. We have to give up ideas about who we wish we were. We have to learn to love ourselves as we are and know that others can love us, too.

Taken as a group, the grasping and healing behaviors act like a big skateboard half-pipe on the playground of your health and wellness. Confusion, resentment, doubt, and fear will ultimately take you down into the dark valley of miserliness and isolation. If, however, you permit yourself to embrace those behaviors and become mindful of their impact, the healing behaviors will then be able to carry you up the other side and out into the light. Committing to awareness, vulnerability, surrender, and authenticity will allow you to form and maintain the connection with yourself and others that will create the joy you were meant to have in your life.

The Mantras

A mantra is a word or phrase that is repeated. Mantras are often used to help focus attention in meditation. In that case, one word or phrase may be expressed over and over throughout the sitting. The mantras developed for use with the Five Tibetan Yogas Workshop will not be repeated over and over again in a single day, but will be repeated each time you do your practice. As such, they are considered to be mantras.

The mantras are your daily connection among the Five Tibetans, the chakras, and the grasping and healing behaviors. I recite the appropriate mantra before I perform each of the Five Tibetans. I then meditate on the mantra when I am in the rest pose. As we move through the workshop, you will learn other meditations and visualizations that will further enhance the essence of each mantra. If these mantras do not parallel your personal spiritual tradition, try creating your own. It is more important that you are developing a contemplative practice than repeating particular words.

The Mantras for the Five
Tibetan Yogas Workshop

The First Tibetan

This is light. Opening the Third Eye. Illuminating darkness, ignorance, confusion, disorientation and panic. Lighting the way for insight and wisdom, clarity and perspective, reality and awareness, acceptance and peace.

The Second Tibetan

This is air. Opening the heart chakra. Blowing away anger and resentment, bitterness, envy, jealousy, animosity, and rage. Creating space for love and compassion, forgiveness and vulnerability, acceptance and peace.

The Third Tibetan

This is fire. Opening the third chakra. The solar plexus. The power center. Burning away frustration, doubt, and shame, ineffectiveness, powerlessness, and grasping. Clearing the way for walking in my divine power and purpose, surrendering to what is, following my guidance, manifesting my dreams, and being at peace.

The Fourth Tibetan

This is water. Opening the belly and sacral chakra. Washing away judgment of myself and others, blame and guilt of myself and others, lack of morality and integrity, smallness and fear. Creating a flow of truth and honor, authenticity, creativity and expansiveness, acceptance and peace.

The Fifth Tibetan

This is earth. Opening the root chakra. Covering inferiority and superiority. Burying arrogance and miserliness. Creating a foundation for oneness, unity, and connection, acceptance and peace.

Part II
Grasping

The Worst Thing I Can Be

*I*have spent a good portion of my life being the thing someone thought was the worst thing imaginable. When I was young, I was very overweight. This was the thing my father thought was the worst thing ("No man will marry you.""No one will love you."). His worst fear was that I would be an unhappy, unmarried woman. I was content to play baseball and build forts in the surrounding meadows, but I received his message loud and clear. What I looked like was not okay.

Later, when I left a marriage and spent my days as an educator with a social conscience, I was two of the worst things my conservative church fellows could imagine: divorced and Democrat. I remember the night before the 1996 election (Clinton vs. Dole), when the church I attended held a dramatic candlelight vigil praying for God's will for the country. God, as it turns out, voted for Clinton. My children were struck with fear knowing that I was not going to vote the way those people wanted me to. They knew what I believed was not okay.

Finally, when I was 42, I announced that I was the thing many people in our American society still believe is the worst thing you can be: I came out as being gay. It is still popular to hate gay folks in this country. It seems to be something many organizations can unite around. I notice the billboards and read the papers and see frequent messages that who I am and who I love are not okay.

I am not sure what I was meant to do with all the input I have received about being the worst thing someone else could imagine. I know that each betrayal by a parent and shunning by a stranger has had an impact. Those hurts and barbs and rejections were like heat-seeking missiles, penetrating my shield of self-protection. They left their dents and stains and destruction. Ignoring their impact only led to my greater impairment. My relationships suffered. I suffered. The inner damage oozed out in my anger and sense of disconnection. Sooner or later, I had to come face to face with more than the memories. I had to have a showdown with the cadavers of all those naysayers of the past. I had to embrace them as being part of *me. It was time to intentionally and mindfully address the parts of my inner life that were wreaking havoc on my outer life.*

It is becoming clearer to me as each year passes that I cannot afford to be the worst thing I can imagine. I have to be able to face all the parts of myself each day and truly believe that I have been created in the image of an infinitely wise and loving God, and that who I am, exactly the way I am, has been created for a purpose: often overweight, Democrat, divorced, and gay—and sometimes confused, resentful, doubtful, afraid, and miserly.

CHAPTER 4

Confusion

This is light.
Opening the Third Eye.
Illumining darkness, ignorance, confusion,
disorientation and panic.

The sun, not rising until well after half-past eight, was a muted orb in the overcast sky. The off-and-on-rain of the past day and night had stopped. Slivers of blue were beginning to show overhead as the dark clouds were teased apart by the coastal breezes. The rainwater that had filled the deep tractor tracks in the field had frozen in the frigid overnight temperatures. The sound of gunshots rang out in the crisp morning air. It was a typical December day in northern Scotland.

I heard the gunfire as I was washing the breakfast dishes. A quick staccato of three or four shots, followed by several hapless singles. I looked at the note posted on the kitchen cabinet door and realized that today was a "shoot," a day when area hunters are permitted to come onto the land and shoot the resident pheasants. It was one of seven such events planned for Saturdays scattered between early November and January. It was going to be a tough day to be a pheasant.

I had become more familiar with pheasants and their habits since arriving at the estate. Distinctively marked with a white band around the neck, glints of red and blue about the head, and brown-striped tail feathers, the pheasant resembles a small, colorful turkey. I think you could go so far as to suggest that pheasants are rather attractive members of the fowl family. Seeing them going about in the garden and on the roads reminded me of the bands of turkeys that used to come marching across my yard when I lived in the hills of Northern California. Unlike their somewhat arrogant California turkey cousins, however, pheasants do not comport themselves in a stately fashion, nor are they oblivious to the habits of man—at least not these particular silly ones, which ran around scared and squawking and wasted no time getting out of the path of an oncoming human. And, today, I understood why. Their home, and mine, could, at any moment, become a war zone.

The game of the day was "beat and shoot." The "beaters," men with big white rectangular fans and bird dogs, went through the fields and woods and shooed the pheasants along. The commotion caused the pheasants to abandon their perches and fly into the air. If the hunters were lucky and the fowl less so, the pheasants would fly up and over the hunters and be shot down.

It was a tough day to be a resident of the estate, too. My plans for a vigorous walk out on the fields and truck routes around the property had been sabotaged. I went out later in the day, hoping they were done with the shoot, for my sake as well as for the benefit of the pheasants. But as I moved out across the rough, golden remnants of cut straw in a field near the cottage, I noticed a line of trucks in the distance, and heard the shots. I retreated.

On my way back to the cottage, I encountered two beaters and their dogs standing in the lane, moving the pheasants from the woods toward the fields that held the hunters I had seen earlier. Two or three of the crazed brown critters ran across in front of me, squabbling their pheasant version of "Oh! No! We are going to die!" Another one flew out of the trees and swooped over me as it headed closer to the woods near the fields. A minute later, I heard the shots.

My assessment as a newcomer to such "sport" is that the primary job of the beaters is to create confusion—a moment of panic that causes the prey to lose its sense of direction and intention and run or fly off toward the hunters. The pheasants would be much better off staying put or flying behind the men bearing the fans, then making a quick retreat in the opposite direction. The beaters, after all, were not the real source of danger. These fowl residents of the estate definitely needed some lessons in self-defense. I laughed to myself as I conjured a vision of a school for pheasants where they were taught how to survive a Saturday shoot. Two pieces of advice for panicky pheasants came immediately to mind: stay put until you have the time to accurately assess your situation, and watch where you fly.

Look Before You Fly

As the afternoon went on, I could not get free of the mental picture of those frightened pheasants running across the road, fleeing from a place of minimal danger and flying right into the outstretched guns of the hunters. My contemplation turned inward, as I considered the times I have tried to escape a minor danger or setback, only to throw myself fully into a much more personally lethal situation. I have a feeling that I am not so different from the pheasants when I am faced with something or someone who "beats" around in my life. A lost job or broken relationship. A lengthy illness. Anything that has the potential to disorient me and send me off course.

Pheasants are not the only ones who struggle with staying put when danger threatens. How often when I see a bad thing coming do I start churning and running around as though flapping my wings and worrying is going to solve the problem? How often do I spin off without even checking to see if there really *is* a problem? Stopping, perhaps winging up into a nearby tree, could be a life-saving move for the pheasants on the day of the estate shoot. The dogs could not reach them. The beaters would move on to find other more cooperative "participants." There they would be, high enough to have some perspective, safe, and in a good place to resume their normal activities once the beaters and dogs had moved on.

Running off in reaction to the danger without taking time to assess its reality and seek perspective is not just fatal for pheasants; it can be destructive for people, too. My boss made an unfair accusation, so I quit. My partner stayed out late after work for the third time this week, so I'll have an affair. My bank account is dwindling, so I am going to lose my house. The mind starts churning, stories are fabricated to substantiate the fears, and soon, we are off and running like a pheasant being shooed from its nest.

It is not easy in times of crisis to sit down and look deeply at what is actually happening, no easier than it would be for a pheasant to slow its wildly pounding little heart, look at a beater, and take a defiant stance. "Really? You expect me to run just because you are flapping your fan?" But I want that for the pheasant. I want to root for the pheasant's ability to take stock and put himself in better stead than he will experience if he is carried along by his fear and instincts. I want better than that for me, too. I tire of reacting every time something or someone causes a ripple in my life.

I have a habit—let's call it a propensity, for honesty's sake—of getting my feelings hurt and then flying off and making some pronouncement. "I don't want to talk with you for a while." "This relationship is not working for me." "I can't do this anymore." Occasionally, my assessment comes after having talked to the other person, but, more likely, I lash out blindly, without getting the full picture, and put the relationship or situation at real risk because I have not looked carefully at what I truly want for myself. The issue here is not whether I allow my feelings to be hurt or that I am disappointed, or angry, or frustrated. That is all normal human fare. The question is, once I am there—steeped in whatever feeling has been accessed—where do I fly?

If you close your eyes, you can see the pheasants in the field. They are walking along awkwardly, as pheasants do, coming upon the beaters and their dogs, feeling confused and afraid. What now? You have wings—why not use them? You take off and, once airborne, have several options. You can fly blindly and get the heck out of there, without thinking of a location that would be safer. You might get lucky and not fly over the hunters. You could also fly to safety—to a familiar tree … to a fat, bushy shrub … to a place where you could rest and reflect and get your bearings.

Pheasants do not have the capacity to contemplate a safe space, but wingless humans do. You can choose a safe haven to run to when you feel mounting confusion and panic. This place is best sorted out in advance of the need to fly. Your office, if private. A park bench. The inside of the car. A walk around the block. A ride up and down the elevator. A meditation cushion. Your special chair. The exact nature of the location will be very personal and will depend on what is available. Knowing your "fly to" place can provide a sense of calm in a brewing emotional storm. And, as you seek a safe space, do it alone. In the first moments of panic or confusion, you are the only person you need to consult. Allow yourself time to be with the situation without adding into the mix the thoughts, words, and emotions of other people.

If In Doubt Just Breathe Out

Like the pheasants, you have evolutionary instincts that click into place ready to assert their own agendas when you face adversity. You are programmed to choose "fight" or "flight," to either defend yourself or run for safety. There are systems in your body that turn on automatically to help you hit harder or run faster. How do you outsmart those diametrically opposed, hard-wired instincts and create another option, a third way, an action somewhere between fighting back and flying away that will allow you to weather the moments of confusion and fear with fewer negative consequences?

If you aren't fighting and you aren't flying away, what is available? Staying, that's what. Remaining present and waiting for what my Quaker friends refer to as "way opening." When you feel yourself whirling and twirling; when your heart is pounding or breaking; when every cell in your body is screaming for you to retreat into isolation; when you are so dizzy from a lack of clarity that you feel you have just been on one of those horrid gravity rides at the fair—really, in times like these, what can you do but stop? And then, once you have stopped, breathe.

I never want it to be that simple. I rebel against the possibility that whatever I am feeling can be transformed by breathing into my belly and out through my mouth. And yet, when I focus on this process, no matter how reluctantly, I am able to regain a sense of myself in the moment. I can feel *me* in the midst of all the confusion and angst.

So, allow yourself time to breathe. Close your eyes. Take a gentle breath in through your nose, and feel the air move down past your diaphragm and fill your belly. Keeping a soft belly is a good indicator of how effective the breath will be. If the belly is soft, the mind and body really have let go. Once you have expanded that nice soft belly, just let the air out gently through your mouth. Stay with your breath. Stop listening to the voices in your head and all the chaos and spinning that is conspiring to take you under. Just breathe. Sooner or later you will feel the sigh come, much like the deep breath an infant takes as she relaxes off into sleep—a deeper in-breath and a fuller out-breath. That sigh is a signal that you have relaxed and are now ready to mindfully ponder the situation.

"But," you ask, "what good is a breath, really? Breathing won't put money in my bank account or resolve a marital affair." Or maybe it will. Perhaps connecting to our center and putting aside all the stories for just a few moments will give us clarity and perspective. Those new insights could then allow us to be grateful for the lessons inherent in the situation and be willing to open ourselves to possibilities, to solutions and resolutions that might not otherwise occur to us. The process reminds me of a line of dominoes, the first one tipping the second and so on down the row. It starts with a breath, which opens a moment of mindfulness. Mindfulness leads to more realistic perceptions. Right perceptions can steer us to gratitude. Once you get to gratitude, you will have effectively transformed the confusion. You will have a higher perspective. You will be able to metaphorically look down on the fields and assess the extent of the danger and decide how you want to be with your circumstances. Now you can see that you have choices. You are free to act rather than react.

Exploring Confusion in the First Tibetan

The First Tibetan beautifully models the process of confusion. As you twirl around, the room moves and objects around you appear in different places. Your relationship to your world shifts. In the process of the spin, you could not just walk over and pick up a book from the table. You would have to stop and orient yourself first, get your balance. A step forward would have to be more deliberate and would likely be somewhat wobbly.

The children's game "Pin the Tail on the Donkey" helps us look at this phenomenon more closely. Remember? You put on the blindfold, confident that you know where everything is and that you will get the paper tail right on the donkey's hindquarters. Your friends, however, are going to give you a little spin first to make it more complicated. By the time they are done with you, you have no idea which way is up, much less where that silly donkey is! You wander around helplessly while everyone is laughing and giving you directions. You have no point of reference to get you anywhere close to the donkey.

I have had some days like that, maybe some years—times when I have been in one spin after another and have had no idea how to get myself where I thought I was going. Taking in random information from people who were trying to help me just made me more confused and disoriented. When you get in a spin in the real world, you will save yourself a lot of time and effort if that first step is a mindful one. You create more possibility by waiting patiently than by impulsively taking off and trying to fix it. The first person who has to clear is you. Give yourself the gift of time.

As you spin around in the First Tibetan, you are creating an imbalance problem that your inner ear has to solve. It is not easy at first. The trick, I think, is in staying with it. By adding two spins each week, little by little, you are decreasing the impact the spin has on your system. It will not be long before you are doing more spins and doing them at a greater speed. This has carry-over to everyday life. As you become more accustomed to handling the spins that life inevitably brings, you will find that while you may still be a little "woozy" in the process, you will come out of it more rapidly.

Light is the transformational element for the First Tibetan. If possible, stop what you are doing right now and complete three spins, so that you can connect with the impact of the light element in the exercise. You may want to practice the mantra before you begin. (*This is light. Opening the Third Eye. Illumining darkness, ignorance, confusion, disorientation and panic. Lighting the way for insight and wisdom, clarity and perspective, reality and awareness, acceptance and peace.*)

If you are willing to risk a bout of vertigo, try doing a few repetitions of the First Tibetan with your eyes closed. Give yourself over to the darkness in your head with no points of reference outside yourself. What do you feel? How does closing out the light impact your ability to be with the spins? For most of us, closing our eyes in the spin would be downright dangerous. We would have no sense of our location with respect to the objects in the room. When you open your eyes, you let the light in. Light is what makes seeing possible. It helps give us a sense of position and direction. You can use this understanding when you are presented with a situation that sends you into emotional turmoil. Find a point of light and allow it to fill the void that has been created by the crisis. Keeping your eyes open, both metaphorically and literally, can lessen the impact of the event facing you.

There are many ways to have points of light at the ready for those moments of impending darkness. Prayer. A favorite song. A poem. I keep a picture of my grandson Ben on the screen of my cell phone. Sometimes by accident, and other times on purpose, I turn on the phone and there he is involved in some sort of antic—feeding his plastic horse macaroni and cheese or stripped to the waist eating dinner with catsup dripping from his fingers or whatever other pose his mother caught him in when she sent me an evening photo. He brings joy into my world. Even a brief moment with his light can open a fissure in whatever darkness I am experiencing. I smile, maybe chuckle out loud, and say, "He is such a cheeky monkey." My heart opens. I breathe in. That moment of mindfulness with the light of my young grandson allows me to get back to the joy of the present. I can then gather myself, say, "Okay, God, I know we can do this thing," and risk another step on the path.

Your practice of the First Tibetan yoga will be followed by Child's Pose. Laying there curled up with your head down you are once again in the fetal position, in the warmth and safety of the womb, folded in, darkness in front of you. Your breath rhythmic and easy. The sound of your heartbeat within your ears. You are a child of the Creator. Your world is a safe place. The spinning has stopped. Stay in the rest pose as long as is necessary to bring you fully back from the spinning. Then, on a day when the spinning has been caused by something in your externalized world, you can come to the mat and rest in the pose until you experience that same calm, until you once again feel safe and steady.

I frequently experience intense emotions in Child's Pose after the First and Fifth Tibetans. Yoga teachers of various traditions have told me this is a common occurrence. I attribute this to the fact that the child in you allows you to be vulnerable, to be open to the feelings of smallness and confusion and pain lodged in your adult body and heart. In Child's Pose, you are free to let it all go. If you feel strong emotions during this time, simply let them surface and have their way. This is part of the process. There will be healing in those tears and cries as some of that "sludge" that has accumulated over the years is released.

In time, as you practice the First Tibetan, you will learn that you can be in the spin, perhaps feel a little dizzy, and yet remain centered and steady when it is over. And so it is in our lives. The spins will come. They are inevitable. If we take time to stop, draw a breath, and be with the feelings rather than let them carry us off squawking and flapping, we have the potential to transform those moments of panic or loss into clarity and awareness.

CHAPTER 5

Resentment

This is air.
Opening the heart chakra.
Blowing away anger and resentment, bitterness,
envy, jealousy, animosity, and rage.

Over the course of my life I have had the "opportunity" to live in tornado alley and hurricane central. I grew up in northeastern Oklahoma where, yes, the wind does literally come sweeping down the plains. In late spring and summer, those winds can become the stuff of violent and destructive tornadoes. Children practice tornado drills at school. The tornado preparedness siren blows in most Oklahoma towns at some point each week. That preparation is important; the average time you have to get to safe shelter is fourteen minutes. Even as I was writing this book, Moore, Oklahoma, was struck by a devastating EF5 tornado that reduced hundreds of homes to matchsticks and destroyed two elementary schools. Seven children were killed in the falling rubble.

Later, in my adult life, I lived in North Carolina. Tropical storms and hurricanes with human names came and went along the coast from June through November every year. I learned the importance of falling into the cultural routine of buying water and basic needs when the weatherman forecasted an approaching storm. Tornadoes and hurricanes share high winds and destruction, but tornadoes have cyclonic winds and hurricanes have straight winds. Another significant difference between these meteorological events is that while you have only minutes to prepare for a tornado, you have days to get your provisions and hunker down for a hurricane. Hurricanes will generally stay longer and impact a larger area. You can be without electricity and water for several days, especially if you live in a rural area.

We had not lived in North Carolina very long when hurricanes Bertha and Fran struck the state in the summer and fall of 1996. My children were young then. We holed up in my upstairs bedroom. (No, we never did that again as one of the main sources of injury in hurricanes is big trees falling on houses.) In both storms, we had very little loss. But during Fran, a nearby neighborhood sustained significant damage. Several houses and cars were smashed by falling trees. Entire sections of roofs were torn off the two-story structures. Soon after the storms had passed, the weatherman reported that the destruction done in that area was due to a tornado. Evidently, tornadoes can be spawned from the thunderstorms that form in the bands of rain around the hurricane. While the raging straight winds of the hurricane did minor damage, the tornado cut a swath of destruction through that neighborhood just a few blocks away from our house.

As we move into a contemplation of the Second Tibetan and its companion grasping behavior, resentment, the picture of little tornadoes of destruction dropping out of the winds of a hurricane was too enticing not to enlist as a parallel. Even better that it follows the "spins" of confusion. Someone has done something to upset your world, has precipitated chaos, discomfort, or self-doubt. You get your feelings hurt. The spin starts. It gains speed and power. Hurt feelings expand. If you do not catch it in time, the pent-up destruction will be unleashed. You will disconnect. You will tell your stories. You will lash out and try to return the pain. If not checked and released, these cyclonic feelings can destroy your friendships, dismantle your partnerships, and extinguish your ability to live compassionately with yourself and others.

A Destructive Pairing

Anger frequently gets top toxicity billing in books about spiritual awakening and healing. While we do not want to hold onto anger, anger is something we are meant to have. Christian scripture instructs its readers to be angry, but to not let the sun go down on the anger (Ephesians 4:26). Bridging those two actions is the admonition to "not sin." The anger is not the "sin"; the hanging onto it is what creates the difficulties. Our anger is part of us and needs to be given due consideration. In *You Are Here*, Thich Nhat Hanh encourages us to be conscious and compassionate about our anger, to refrain from splitting it off and denouncing it as something bad in us. He teaches us to hold our anger close and acknowledge it with an actual expression of connection. For example, you might say, "Dear anger, I see that you are in me, and I am here for you."

The danger with anger is not that we have it, but that we may not choose to release it. We might decide to allow it to hang around and mature. I lived in France long enough for this to conjure the whiff of an overripe cheese in my olfactory memory. The thing that was good at one time has outlived its usefulness and is spreading a foul odor; it now has a life of its own. It seems to be the same with anger and resentment. We feed anger with our doubts and fears. We create stories about the insult and injury we experienced. The resentment becomes a self-righteous retreat for our own feelings of smallness and inferiority. If we are not mindful, we become prone to all the maladies of body and spirit that thrive in the twisters of these negative emotions. Sore backs. Headaches. Isolation. Vengeance. Even chronic and fatal diseases have been attributed to the biochemical disturbances that can manifest when anger is left to brew.

Anger is not the enemy. It signals us that we need to be in action—perhaps moving away from something that is not in our best interest, perhaps moving toward a change that we are resisting. Anger, in and of itself, is a healthy emotion. Resentment, on the other hand, has the power to suck the life out of us and the people around us.

For the purpose of writing this chapter, I spent time researching the origins and definition of the word "resentment." You might be surprised to discover that the word "resent" is derived from a Latin precursor that meant, literally, to "refeel." When we are resenting someone or something, we are actually re-feeling the hurts and pains and disappointments that have come before; we are living in the past. Unfortunately, we are also impacting the present and setting ourselves up for problems in the future.

For the purpose of our discussion I created a working definition for resentment by blending entries from two dictionary sources: *Resentment is indignation or persistent ill will as a result of a real or imagined wrong, insult, or injury.* The key words in this rendering of resentment are, for me, "persistent" and "imagined." That is the crux of it, really. In order to enter into the bowels of resentment, you have to latch onto a perceived hurt and declare by your words and actions that you will not be shaken from your pole. In so doing, you grasp onto something absolutely undesirable. It is a dangerous place to be. At best you will distance yourself from one person who has inflicted a real or imagined hurt; at worst, you set yourself up for an ever-growing list of people you feel justified to cut off from your love and your life.

Uncovering Resentment

How do we keep our imaginations from creating situations of persistent ill will? As I was writing this book, I found that I was working around this chapter, moving on to Doubt and Fear, creating outlines for the healing behaviors, not feeling drawn to the topic, not seeing in-my-face natural lessons out there just waiting to be wrestled into a chapter about resentment. I thought, "Hmm, I must not be meant to write the Resentment chapter right now. Maybe that is not what needs attention in my life right now. I feel happy. I am enjoying where I am in my life."

Some of you are already laughing.

I want to stop right here and say that I have found that this is a critical problem with resentment. It can be a seething monster that stalks our consciousness and looks back at us from the mirror every morning. But I think it more frequently exists at a deeper level, under the surface, lurking in the shadows of our hearts. Little twisters of persistent ill will just waiting to be unleashed to threaten our relationships and our own well-being. I have become increasingly sensitive to what may really be behind someone telling me he is in a "good place" and is not needing to deal with this person or that situation.

Let me say gently, and rather emphatically, if you are cutting yourself off from the people around you (except in situations where safety is involved, of course), you are probably not "in a good place." You might have found a safe hole to curl up in to delay taking out your resentment entourage and looking at it, but I imagine you are feeling some backlash from your choice. Time? Energy? Isolation? More hurt feelings? No worries. It will all be there when you really do get "in a good place" and decide to take a look. It will just be bigger and gooier then.

Before you start thinking I am getting a little too big for my britches to be making that strong a statement, let me share the rest of my story about "finding" resentment as I was writing the book. Without going into too much detail, I began to be aware of several examples of places where I was harboring persistent ill will for real or imagined injuries to my person. I noticed that there were times when the name or thought of this person or that person would bring out several sentences related to my hurt feelings. Generally, there would be a barb or two back at them in there, too. Then, we were planning an event at The Lodge in France. We had created a guest list. A few years earlier, I had had a slight run in with one of the people on the list. I could feel my desire to consider not asking that person to participate. I could feel myself prepping for a confrontation. I could feel ill will three years later. I was aware of a sense of real or imagined personal injury sitting in there, under the surface, like an ancient rock from the Grampian Mountains resting at the bottom of the cold North Sea. Three years later, here it comes rolling back onto the shore to be reckoned with.

Opening myself to what was happening in the situation in France made me hyper-aware of other situations where I was holding something against someone else. Among the lot were a parent, a former partner, a sister, and a friend. Rather the gamut of possibilities, don't you think? Nothing vicious; some no big deal— but a collection was brewing, a group of people whose past deeds were being "re-felt" in my present.

Grasping comes in all shapes and sizes. We often picture it as the desire to hold onto something good that is being taken away from us. But we can also grasp at things we should and need to let go of. Here, grasping is more clinging, like a child might latch onto a filthy old stuffed animal that needs to be laid to rest. Why do we do it? Why do we want to hold onto the hurtful words or actions that others might send our way? A relationship ends. Why do we cling to the bitter bits? A parent says something hurtful. Why do we let that find its way inside of us? A friend steps away in our time of need. A stranger embarrasses us. How can it possibly serve me to hold onto past offenses?

As adults, we tend to hang onto our "childish things." I believe that early in our lives resentment may have been a self-protective behavior we developed before we were able to take care of ourselves. If someone was "mean" or "hurtful," we learned to shut ourselves off from her or avoid him as a means of protecting ourselves. If someone disappointed us time and time again, we stopped depending on her. It makes sense … when you are four or eight years old. But protecting ourselves by "going away" from the people who hurt us is not such a sensible behavior when we are fully grown, functioning adults. That self-protective response is now a sign of our inability or unwillingness to open our hearts to others in love and compassion, to step fully into our own power, to be vulnerable and authentic, to release the victim mentality and assume the posture of a grounded and responsible grownup. Yes, there are some advantages to being just eight.

Obviously, this chapter had to wait to be written until all the characters of my little resentment party were in place. At least, I hope these were all the characters. The dance floor was getting pretty crowded. This is another of the insidious characteristics of resentment. Once we let ourselves begin the process, the goo from one held hurt creates an attachment for another imagined slight, and soon we are carrying around an awkward conglomerate of our perceived worst parts of the past.

Do you have a list, too? Maybe I should start by asking if you are hiding from the list, too. It is difficult to face both the wounds that have been rendered and the people who have allegedly inflicted them. We need to look deeply at these things when they first occur. But it just feels easier—and safer—to walk away, to hide out, to isolate, and to let the little splinters of hurt and disappointment fester out of sight.

As I came to grips with my own list, I noticed that I had certain "tells" that would signal me that I had gone to that place of holding ill will. First, I became aware that I could not make eye contact. I am generally a look-you-in-the-eye-and-shake-your-hand kind of person. I assume I avoid the eyes of the other person because I either do not want her to see the hurt or disappointment in me or I do not want to see the Divine in him. I look away or down or to the side rather than taking the object of my resentment in by the seat of the soul. Second, I distance physically. I will not choose to have a conversation with him. I prefer not to sit next to her. I want a physical distance to create a buffer between the person and what I am holding back. We will get to miserliness a little later on, but you can already see the withholding begin to take shape. Withdrawing my emotional connection, my physical presence, and my affection are ways of cutting myself off and not having to deal with what I am feeling.

Exploring Resentment
Using the Second Tibetan

Whew! There is a lot on the table right now. If you know that there are resentments brewing inside you, you might be feeling overwhelmed, and if you are insisting there are no resentments brewing inside you, you might be thinking you need to move onto a different chapter. This is the place in a workshop where your facilitator would ask you to "do" something. To allow the energy to move. So, I will ask you to get down on the floor, if at all possible, and do the Second Tibetan. If you are following along with the 12-week plan, this is a great time to become very familiar with the mantra for the Second Tibetan and to let its meaning move in your body with the flow of the pose. (*This is air. Opening the heart chakra. Blowing away anger and resentment, bitterness, envy, jealousy, animosity, and rage. Creating space for love and compassion, forgiveness and vulnerability, acceptance and peace.*)

As you start the pose, notice any tightness or restriction in your breathing. Contemplate that the representative element for the Second Tibetan is air. Air has the capacity to seep into places that are shut off. Think of how difficult it is to create an air-tight house in the winter. Air also invigorates and brings freshness. Air, by its very nature as a gas, is expansive. It is more than fluid. It can be everywhere at once. Air is susceptible to the laws of diffusion and will always move from a place where there is more of it to a place where there is less.

As you now perform the Second Tibetan, inhale as you lift your hips off the floor and move your chest upwards. Visualize your heart and chest being full of air, opening as the expansiveness of the gas takes up more and more space. What needs to be pushed out? Let those things go as you breathe out and return to the resting position. I encourage you to perform at least three repetitions of the pose.

In each case, be mindful of your thoughts and feelings. Is there anger? Hurt? Sadness? Are the tears making their way to the corners of your eyes? Can you breathe easily or is the breath stiff and ragged? You do not need to do anything with these observations. Notice. Move on.

Once you have completed the three repetitions of the Second Tibetan, I invite you to rest in Corpse Pose. Corpse is an apt name for what can occur in your life and relationships if you do not release the death and destruction resentment can bring into your heart. It is also a picture of giving up those persistently held hurts and hard feelings. Let them die. Allow them to make their way back into the earth and become compost to feed the thoughts and actions of a higher calling. As you take complete breaths (see Chapter 1), visualize a warm breeze blowing over your body—the kind of breeze you might feel when you are lying on the beach, sun shining down on your face, perhaps a little damp from taking a swim. As you remain in Corpse Pose, let that movement of air over your body take the resentment and held hurts in its delicate tendrils and carry them away. As the breeze moves over you, think or say aloud the names and events you are holding, acknowledging that they are keeping you small and unable to move freely and confidently in your world. As the breeze makes each pass, keep releasing those names and specific events until no more surface. Take a moment to deeply breathe and feel the air expand your heart, opening you to compassion and forgiveness. Feel the lightness the release has brought. Take a moment to offer gratitude for the people and situations you have named.

If you are following along with the 12-week program, repeat the meditation each time you do the Second Tibetan during the week. Each day, use your journey journal to record the names and events that you give up to the breeze. As the week progresses, note any shifts in your thoughts or actions toward the people and situations on your list. To aid in the process, offer gratitude for the people on your list each day as part of your practice this week.

CHAPTER 6

Doubt

This is fire.
Opening the third chakra, the solar plexus, the power center.
Burning away frustration, doubt, and shame,
ineffectiveness, powerlessness, and grasping.

It was one of the colder January mornings in the French Alps that winter. I awoke to the sound of the harp alarm on my iPhone, a sense of dread immediately spreading over me like the cold, frozen fog that descends on the mountain valley. I could feel resistance starting in my head and moving like lightning all the way down to my soon-to-be-in-ski-boots feet. I was scheduled for a ski lesson at Les Deux Alpes, the resort that watches over the Lodge from its heights on the nearby mountain.

I am relatively certain that if you look up the phrase "world's biggest, slippy, slidey chicken" in the record book you would find a picture of me, sitting or standing with a look on my face that would match the pheasant's expression on shooting day. I am not really sure why. But I hate (and yes, I know, hate is a four-letter word), I *hate* the feeling of my feet slipping out from under me. I need more control than that. But, I also do not enjoy everyone else going off on a day to ski and leaving me to sit home. I feel left out when the conversation turns to this piste and that run and whatever ski lingo happens to come at the time. So, I decided while I was once again in France in the winter, I would have a go at putting on skis and learning how to actually play with them. Although from my perspective, it was akin to inviting a vicious, blood thirsty animal bent on my destruction over for a play date. Like I said… hate it.

As I prepared for my little adventure, I did one of each of the Five Tibetans, performing each pose slowly and methodically, hoping some of the attributes I claim for them would stick with me. I could feel my heart pounding in my chest.

When the inevitable time arrived, my friend drove me to the *téléphérique* at nearby Venosc. I got out of the car and began my solitary ascent to the top of the mountain. I bought a ticket for the ride up, got into one of the little go-up-and-down-cars, and was suspended in the air a hundred feet off the ground, watching the top of the mountain come toward me. I was fine during the ride. It was really beautiful scenery, and the sun was just striking the snowy tops of the mountains that surrounded me. It was also scary enough to take my mind off the lesson.

I arrived at the top and walked to the *location* (a French ski rental shop) where I had been told to get my skis and meet the teacher. I got outfitted, then had 30 minutes to wait. I sat on the bench at the back of the shop and meditated, trying to get my heart beat down to a rate that might not lead to a coronary in the middle of the lesson. I talked to myself. I prayed. I gave myself a short Reiki session and did affirmations.

Way too soon my teacher arrived, selected another pair of skis for me that she liked better, and we set off for "the Baby Snow" (it's true, that is its name). We took the free button lift that carries *debutantes* (there were three-year-olds on this slope): it was a short distance up the hill, so that they can learn to ski down. The chapter on vulnerability is coming up. This could have gone in that slot, too.

I *was* feeling vulnerable. I was afraid of looking silly. I was afraid of falling down. I was afraid of being sprawled out on the ground and not able to get up. As the morning progressed, all those fears would, sooner or later, be realized.

When we walked onto the snow on the piste, the teacher told me to put on my skis. I was personally thinking that the snow looked pretty good for treading farther on foot. She was, however, insistent. I followed her instructions and put on the skis, clutching to my sticks for dear life. "Stand up straight," she said. "Head up. Legs forward against your boots." Any one of those instructions would have been difficult, but as a set? You have to be kidding. Look up? Trust my skis? When I did look up, though, the beauty of bright blue sky and mountain backdrop was worth the effort. And then that slippy-slidey thing happened, and I tensed up to resist the possibility of a header onto the snow.

We walked across the wee *piste*. The teacher taught me to traverse a ridge, snow-plow to control my speed, and turn my head to turn my body. Any time I gathered any speed, I would panic and flail my sticks, once almost sending both of us rolling down the hill as my sticks got under her right ski. It was the only time she got agitated with me. I finally got down the hill, and the teacher directed me toward the lift for the Baby Snow. This lift did not have chairs. Instead you straddled a round metal plate (button) attached to a pole and were pulled up the hill on a rotating cable. I skied into the queue, and we rode up together on the buttons just like the moms riding beside their toddlers. The teacher helped me get off at the top. We skied down again, where, as she said later, I freaked out a little less.

Now it was time for me to get off the lift by myself. The three-year-olds were doing it. There was a gang of six-year-olds doing it. I should be able to do this. Stand up straight. Keep your skis apart. Don't sit down on the button. Take it out from between your legs when you get to the hump at the top. Let go and ski to the side so you won't get plowed down by the next button-rider. Simple.

The first time I went solo, I got the round plate out from between my legs, but held onto the pole too long and got dragged a bit before I could extract myself and get my balance. Good try. We went down the hill and back into the line for the lift. This time, as we were being dragged up the hill, I spied a group of preteens in a ski school group led by a girl in a hot pink coat heading right for the exit point of the lift. My teacher had gone in front of me and, as I approached the release point, she started yelling at the group, who stopped just shy of the place I was to dismount. I held onto the button pole. My teacher started screaming, "Let go! Let go!" I finally did, but was afraid of running into the kids and went down in a heap, my right ski disengaging. The teacher got me up and gave me a pep talk. Next time will be better.

We went around the circuit one more time, and I was really psyched to get the lift issue licked. I would let go earlier. I would ski gracefully over to the side. I was set. When I got to the top, I pulled the button out from between my legs and prepared to let go, but the lift pole jerked and I went down head first with my legs spread apart under me and the toe of each ski set firmly in the snow. Fortunately, there was no one behind me ... because *my* behind was straight up in the air in the center of the exit point. The teacher calmly got me sorted out and said, "Now you know how to get up when you fall like that."

I called it a day after we got down the hill. My heart was not into another try on the lift. At that point, I no longer believed I could make it happen. I was not up for another up-ender or face plant. The offered *chocolat chaud* was a welcome relief.

After I got home and relived the events, I had to consider whether I would go again. I tried visualizing myself being hauled by the lift up to the hump that signaled the end, smoothly dismounting and letting go, and skiing over to the side. But I realized that I had no idea what that would *feel* like. All I knew was how it felt to fall, to be anxious, to lose my balance. The doubt that sent me on my face twice that day started to work its way into the story I was telling about me and skiing. I can't get off the lift. I always fall down. I don't think I want to do this again. *Why* would I want to do this again?

I really wanted to learn to be able to ski a little. I went in with great resolve, but the heart palpitations alone were a good indicator that part of me was working against the plan. I had tried skiing before. Always ended up on my back or face sooner or later. I hated the feeling of speed. My story went something like this, "I cannot ski because I cannot get off the lifts." I carried a deep-seated skepticism into the process. As I learned on my attempts to get off the lift, no amount of visualizing can overcome a truckload of doubt.

The Trouble with Doubt

Doubt is a source of great disablement. It has the capacity to dampen your life spark and destroy your relationships. In our analysis of the downward pull of the grasping behaviors, doubt naturally follows confusion and resentment. You get spun by a person or an event. You grasp and hold your hurt feelings. Now, you have a decision to make: Are you willing to let go and walk with confidence and faith in the midst of difficulties and disagreements? Or do you get stuck in an internal battle for control and self-appeasement?

Doubt is a word we use all the time. "I doubt it," we say, when someone asks us if we are going to do something that we are not sure about. "I don't doubt it," we respond, when we hear something that is not surprising to us. What does it really mean to doubt? Most of us tend to use the word to denote a lack of confidence in something or a belief that something may not be true. The etymology of the word doubt, however, indicates that it is more about hesitating or wavering when we have to choose between two things than about signifying we feel uncertain about something. Doubt is the emotional or analysis paralysis we can experience when we stand at a crossroad in our life or our relationships.

I first learned this connotation for doubt when I was reading *The Great Work of Your Life*, Stephen Cope's analysis of Arjuna's struggle in the *Bhagavad Gita*. In his discussion of a warrior's dilemma, Cope tells us that although Eastern contemplative traditions frequently position grasping as the primary torment in the human realm, doubt is the chief affliction of people of action. Doubt creates a sense of being stuck when we cannot find our way to one side or the other of two contradictory propositions. It is "being in two minds at once" or "double minded." In Arjuna's case, doubt and grasping were enemies of his dharma. His life purpose was put at risk by his reluctance to choose to step into his higher calling.

Our interest in this two-edged sword called doubt is not specifically in the context of our exploring our life's purpose; we are more concerned with the inward reckoning that will take us either on a road up and out of the spiral of grasping or will send us perilously closer to disconnection. Calling on what we learned about the chakras in Chapter 2, we know doubt emanates from an unbalanced third chakra, the solar plexus. When we are mired in doubt, we are not stepping forward decisively. We are not trusting ourselves. That lack of confidence suggests a diminished vitality in our purpose and power. When our sense of personal power is askew, we are less likely to be able to take on the imperfections we experience in ourselves or our fellow humans. I am beginning to think of doubt as a self-made purgatory constructed by our inability to step fully into our own divine power and purpose or to acknowledge the same in those around us. It is the epitome of emotional "stuckness."

Some of the most persistent memories of my winter ski lesson adventures were the several times I found myself on some little hump or other, ski tips together, sitting back in my boots, looking down the mountain, and being totally motionless, stuck, unable to move forward, not trusting the skis or my teachers or myself. As I have analyzed those moments from a distance now, I am reminded of a rule of physics: an object at rest will stay at rest unless acted on by an unbalanced force.

When I was stuck standing on my skis, there were two forces at work inside me. One was a strong sense of "I want to do it"; the other was an equally powerful belief that "I cannot do it." When neither of those forces rises to the top to create an imbalance in its direction, motion is impossible. I could not move until the "I want to do it" force was great enough to overcome the inertia of the "I cannot do it" force. It was a miserable and frustrating place to be. In one case, I recall a friend saying to me in a loving, but exasperated way, "You can stand there sitting back in your boots or you can do what you came here to do." In other words, stop holding yourself back from what you came here to accomplish.

The stalemate that resulted in my lack of motion was an indication that I did really want to do it. Otherwise, I would have simply removed my skis and walked down the hill. Equally true was the fact that if I had believed I could do it, I would have set my ski tips parallel to one another and gone off down the slope. In those moments of paralysis there was a battle going on. Neither side was winning. The combination of the two opposing forces, or beliefs, left me standing and watching while everyone else was skiing past me. That is a poignant picture of what can also happen to us in life and relationships. We are standing there stuck in one place, while love and possibility swirl around us.

Resistance and Insistence

When doubt comes to visit it is frequently accompanied by two of its most mischievous associates: resistance and insistence. When you find yourself in a standoff of doubt, you might be asking yourself, "How can I make myself do this?" Making ourselves do something is frequently a precursor to failure or disaster. As I have contemplated the concept of doubt and its impact on my relationship with myself and others, I have been learning that the key to resolution is to simply ask, "Am I resisting or insisting?" That question shifts everything. It will no longer be about what is happening around you. You will lay aside your old stories and whatever hurt or irritation is in the moment as you begin to explore your own part in the event.

Remembering those motionless moments at the top of the hill and my inability to get gracefully off the lift, I am certain I was resisting—the speed, the possibility of a fall, looking silly. If I had been willing to fall and look ridiculous, I would have just gone for it, thought nothing of it. My resistance against what might happen kept me from experiencing what could happen. Yes, I could fall. Yes, I could also ski off with no mishap. Both were equally true. Allowing for the possibility of the fall was the only way I was going to experience the joy of cleanly dismounting from the lift or skiing down the hill.

Resistance is another force in the doubt system. We can think of it as being the friction that holds us tightly in our stuck place. Visualize trying to slide a brick down a hill made of Styrofoam. It just is not going to happen. The brick is going to sink in and, short of tearing up your pretty incline, will not be moveable.

How does that relate to our relationships? When we refuse to forgive someone or let a negative situation go, when we are stuck in our resentment, what possibility are we ignoring as we resist offering unconditional love and acceptance? I was recently in a place where I was feeling consistently at odds with a person I was dealing with every day. I could see it happening, but I was not sure how I was going to shift it. Through my work in meditation and daily practice, I could see that I was resisting almost everything that was in my space. I was not trying to transform the situation or consider the gifts in it. All I could focus on was wanting to be done and gone. A popular coaching adage applies here, "What you resist persists." The more I resisted, the worse things got. The two of us just dug ourselves deeper into the mud and muck of hurt feelings and frustration.

Every doubt has a kernel of goodness. That is the logical conclusion of being torn between two opposites: there can be no doubt without the presence of contrasting beliefs. If it is "all bad," or if you believe the situation is unredeemable, you will give up, take off your proverbial skis, and walk away. I find this very encouraging. It tells me that one path on the doubt crossroad leads to peace and restoration; I just have to find out what that is. When you are feeling stuck and having doubts, take time to be mindful about the good news the doubt is bringing you. What are you being moved toward? Explore your resistance more carefully. What are your beliefs? If you let go and move, what amazing possibilities might show up? At times, our resistance can be a sign that we simply do not feel ready to take the next big step. It may be that we are aware that the workload or our level of commitment will have to increase.

Try a similar strategy when you doubt the intentions of a person who has hurt you. Take time to examine why you are experiencing doubt in the first place. There must be a reason for you to be torn in your thinking. If there is negative, there is almost certainly a positive. Moving slightly toward the more constructive side of your doubt may bring about an enormous shift in the situation. You will tilt the balance in favor of a peaceful resolution.

Resistance is frequently a passive response to a situation. Silence and distancing can be indicators that resistance is being applied. Insistence, on the other hand, is rarely passive or silent. Insistence is pushing and pulling, generally in the direction of your will; it is often the aggressive side of the doubting dilemma. Insistence may show up in your doubting moment as a need to have the situation resolve itself by your prescription—your way or the highway, so to speak. In more extreme cases, insistence can show up as "power over" others, often an indication that excessive energy in the third chakra is in need of balancing.

I think there is a tendency to see passive resistance as a more noble response than aggressive insistence. After all, if you are simply resisting, you may not be saying or doing anything. I wish I were built as a resistor, but I must confess that I tend to be an insister. If I am in a bad place personally, I verbalize about what is happening to me rather than sit silently on the sidelines. In a stuck place, I am the one who gets loud. I have experienced shame around that part of my personality.

I found a bit of clarity and relief when I read *Crucial Conversations*. In this book about successful strategies for having difficult conversations, the authors contend that both "silencing" and "violencing" (their versions of resisting and insisting) are ineffective measures for relieving conflict and creating positive relationships. Whether you drop out of a situation or charge in, you are not contributing authentic input or acting in integrity. Both strategies have the power to kill communication and put the future of the relationship at risk. When resisting or insisting, we are attempting to move the scale to our side of the situation. It is about me, not about we. We are not considering the bigger picture of what may be in our best interest—or the best and highest interest of the other person—in the long run.

Looking Into Doubt with the Third Tibetan

If you are able, I invite you to take time out now to do three repetitions of the Third Tibetan to lock in the learning from this chapter. When you are ready, kneel down and place your hands on your lower back. Begin by repeating the mantra to be mindful of the work that is before you in this pose. (*This is fire. Opening the third chakra. The solar plexus. The power center. Burning away frustration, doubt, and shame, ineffectiveness, powerlessness, and grasping. Clearing the way for walking in my divine power and purpose, surrendering to what is, following my guidance, manifesting my dreams, and being at peace.*)

Inhale as your open your chest and pull your "wings" back. Lean back into the pose. Your chest and shoulders will expand. Your solar plexus will thrust upward to meet the heavens. Your throat will be vulnerable and exposed as your head moves gently back. Let yourself be fully with the movements and the meanings of the pose. By opening yourself you are acknowledging your own power and strength. You know that you are capable of dealing with anything that comes your way. You are able to transform doubt into compassionate knowing.

When you are ready, return to the starting position and exhale. In that breath, release anything that is holding back your ability to stride confidently into your world. Is there shame? Frustration? Grasping? Are you feeling ineffective or powerless? You may want to exaggerate your exhalations to emphasize the release of the thoughts and behaviors that are keeping you from accomplishing your highest purpose.

One of my secrets about my ski school adventure is that the "hump" that was making my life so miserable at the end of the lift run was no more than a meter high. There was no mountain. No hill. Just a hump. A little run up when you are on the button and a little slide down once you get off. How many times have I been stumped by a hump of some sort or other? How often do I let a little doubt send me flying into a heap?

The element associated with the Third Tibetan is fire. What better tool to melt away that hump of doubt than a nice hot flame? Today, as you move into Child's Pose after your repetitions of the Third Tibetan, I invite you to meditate on the flame that is alight within you. Feel the warmth and the power of it. Set an intention that any barriers to you being a confident warrior in your own life will be brought to your mind. As each one comes, visualize it as a lump of snow or ice and place it in the flame. Watch it melt away. As each lump that has represented a doubt is transformed, say to yourself, "I am free of_____."

Consider doing this meditation each day for a week to allow time and opportunity for a deep cleansing of the doubt that is hindering your life and your relationships. Commit to being honest with yourself and not shying away from anything that comes to you in those moments. If you are keeping a journey journal, I encourage you to write down what you melt in the fire of your own flame each day. This will help you be more conscious of the areas of your being and doing that are healing in the midst of your practice.

Final Thoughts

A week or so after my first ski lesson, a friend of mine who is an expert skier took me back to the Baby Snow. We practiced going down a hill. We never went to the lift. I decided not to make the day be about getting over the hump; I wanted to learn how to trust the skis. At one point my friend directed me to go down a steep part of the hill and cut to the left by only turning my head and looking in that direction. I started down the hill and everything in my mind was screaming, "Do not do this!" The doubt machine was telling me it would not work, while my belief in my friend's expertise assured me that it would. I could literally feel a war breaking out in my limbs as some internal mechanism was violently trying to get me to snow plow my way to safety. But I kept my head and body turning to the left. My sticks remained down at my sides. I didn't flail or freak. I let the skis do their work. I trusted my friend. I trusted me. I made it to the other side.

CHAPTER 7

Fear

This is water.
Opening the belly and sacral chakra.
Washing away judgment of myself and others,
blame and guilt of myself and others, lack of morality
and integrity, smallness and fear.

It was a beautiful Saturday afternoon in May, Memorial Day weekend in America. The sky was cloudless, blue, and bright. The high humidity and temperatures that left us feeling like damp sponges a week before had receded. It was truly a perfect late spring day.

I was leading the inaugural Five Tibetans Workshop Preview at a yoga studio in North Carolina. I had booked a full workshop there for the fall and wanted to generate curiosity and interest before I left to go to France for the summer. I was excited to see the dream begin to take form: a *workshop* on the schedule, a chance to share my passion and vision about creating a life-changing daily personal practice around the Five Tibetans.

Five people had signed up for the event, a good number for such a grand day on a holiday weekend. As it turned out, in addition to myself, there were eight participants, including veteran yoga teachers representing the Hatha traditions. It was one of those teachers who had originally believed that the studio owner was bringing in five Tibetan monks to teach the poses. We all joked about the notion that five robed monks might have shown up to teach the class. I laughed and said, "No, nothing special or exotic. Just me—a middle-aged Caucasian woman." That "confession" allowed a sense of smallness and "not-enoughness" to creep into my consciousness. Who am I to share an ancient Tibetan rite that I learned from a

Reiki Master/Teacher in northern Scotland? Really? Who do I think I am? (Translation: *I am afraid they will think I am a fraud.*)

I am not sure exactly when I succumbed to the intimidation and insecurity that I felt. I know I spoke it more than once, putting out into the space that I was uncomfortable teaching what could be considered yoga to yoga teachers. Not only was I not a yoga teacher, I was barely a yoga student. I had just in the two weeks prior to the workshop begun to delve into Hatha yoga, learning *asanas* to get a feel for how yoga is taught in a studio setting.

I do not recall ever having such a rough start in a presentation. That is saying a lot considering I have 30-plus years of teaching, presenting papers and workshops, and facilitation behind me. I had too much material for our short time. I was too intense as I shared my passion for the subject. Rather than just let the Five Tibetans do their work, my story and message got in the way. I was too aware of what I did not know to let what I did know shine through. In the end I "outed" myself and my friend, confessed to stripping half-naked to do the Fifth Tibetan, and lost control of the group during the preliminary stretches. I felt like a student teacher on her first day with a class of 30 ninth graders. (You can only truly appreciate that analogy if you have ever stood in front of a class of thirty14-year-olds.)

There was a palpable discomfort. At one point, a friend of mine stopped participating in the activities and beamed Reiki at me. The wheels were riding on the edge of the axle. Simply being with the knowledge of the yoga teachers surrounding me would have been challenge enough, but I was also very uncomfortable with the form of "spirituality" I had brought to share.

I was leading this workshop preview in the Bible Belt, heralding a message that would have been considered "dark" in my days in the conservative churches of the area. I became overly concerned with what some of the participants were thinking or feeling and made too much of the possibility of our differences rather than just delivering the message of love I had been given. I made apologies. My heart beat wildly and my throat tightened as I spoke the guided meditation to ground, center, and protect: connecting to Source, grounding ourselves by attaching to our own special crystal at the center of Mother Earth, and setting up pyramids of protection. In my mind, I was thinking it had all the makings of a Sunday morning sermon built on what happens when we let the devil into our hearts.

I left feeling embarrassed and disappointed in myself. I was afraid that I had alienated the participants from wanting to engage further with the Five Tibetans. Rather than inspire and ignite their interest, I felt I had asked them to drink from a fire hose and watch a train wreck. I made it through and heard the voice in my head say, "It's not how you start, but how you end that they will remember." I had the knowing that if I was that afraid of offering the meditation, the message must need to go out into the space for someone there. I stayed in the process, tried to hide my humiliation as best I could, and got out alive.

The Fear Factor

When I initially planned this chapter, I assumed it would begin with some adventure tale based on my experience with physical peril—a "real fear" event that would serve as an apt metaphor to lock in the learning. But fear comes to us in many forms, and while there are still places in the world today where people live in actual fear for their personal safety, I would venture to say that most of us rarely experience real physical danger or calamity. Instead, we live in fear of other things. Rejection. Embarrassment. Powerlessness. Humiliation. Lack of control. Failure. Being thought a fool. These are the dangers of our enlightened Western culture. Several of them were working on me that day in the yoga studio.

The fear of what others will think, or are thinking, is a kind of death. It kills our creativity and our best intentions, and it kills possibility. I heard a teacher once say that fear immobilizes and faith empowers. I was immobilized that day in the yoga studio, like the proverbial deer in the headlights. My joy in sharing something I love to do each day was derailed by my fear that I was not good enough to deliver the message, that the message would be offensive, and that, as a result, I and my beloved practice would be seen as imposters.

Fear often comes packaged with its equally nefarious teammate, judgment. Stirring together fear of being judged and judging ourselves is a recipe for disaster … and disappointment … and discouragement. We may become too willing to just slink away and nurse our wounds and tell ourselves that we are not the right person for the job. If we let that inner critic seduce us, we cannot accomplish our purpose. When I let myself be taken over by a fear of what the participants would think about my meditation practice, I was at once judging their response and afraid of it. My fear of their judgment threatened to shut me down entirely.

After spending some time contemplating my experience with the yoga teachers, I realized that I had forgotten the main rule of teaching. I had lost sight of the fact that no matter what the audience brought with them, I was the expert on the topic I was presenting. No one there knew more about the Five Tibetans than I did. That is why they came that day. My audience was going to take my lead. If I exuded confidence, they were going to have confidence in me. If I let out the scent of fear and insecurity, they were going to question my authority. I had fogged the room with my own debilitating fear.

Fear can be your enemy and your friend. It can push you into action to avoid devastation (like being hit by a semi) or it can steal your energy and send you into lifelessness. Knowing when fear is lurking in the shadows is essential to your ability to address its presence and effects. The essence of fear is the perception that we are at risk. That our safety (physical or psychological) is in jeopardy. In *Shaman, Healer, Sage*, Villoldo tells us that South American shamans consider fear to be the greatest enemy. Like the lethal, quiet stalkers of the night jungle, fear is an elusive opponent. It will entice you to engage, but in so doing you will be torn limb from limb; you cannot emerge the victor. You will lose or give up something in the process.

You are best suited to deal with an intruder when you know who or what it is. You are not going to take the same action when a raccoon breaks into your house at night as you are when an armed thief comes through the door. You need to be able to identify fear when it appears. Fear comes knocking dressed as many things, among them are worry, anxiety, doubt, and anger. If you are able to recognize fear for what it is, you can more easily transform your reaction to the situation.

Stepping into Fear

Fear is another word we use in a variety of situations. If you listen closely to the random conversations in your day, you will hear people confess to being afraid of everything from a winter weather forecast to the rising price of gasoline. We use the word "fear" ubiquitously as a way to express our uneasiness with the events going on around us that we cannot control. Frequently, the discomforts are all in our minds and are never realized.

The word fear was originally associated with the presence of danger or calamity; there was no emotion implicit in the word. The notion of fear being a reaction to danger evolved much later in the etymology of the word. I found this fact interesting to ponder. Originally the fear was "out there," and now the fear is "in here." Indeed, more often than not, the fear we conjure is entirely "in here." We are reacting to our perception, rather than the reality, of danger or calamity.

If you said to a friend today that you were feeling fear, he could probably name the symptoms you were experiencing. The heat or churning in the belly. The shortness of breath. The tightness in the chest. The need to run and hide or escape the situation. The physical response to fear is universal; it is dictated by the organs and the chemicals in our body. While our existence has become more mundane over time (compared to the possibility of being eaten alive by a wild animal), the list of physiological responses we know as fear has remained relatively unchanged.

Another less referenced response to fear is "freeze." In the animal world, freeze is an adaptive response that provides for the possibility of the animal's survival when the odds of winning a fight or escaping are low. Once the animal has determined that it cannot fend off the attacker, an array of shock reflexes will set in. The animal will drop to the ground and "play dead." The respiration will abate dramatically. The blood pressure will plummet. The body will either become stiff or malleable like modeling clay (i.e., stay where it is moved). One of the more fascinating aspects of the shock reflex is that the animal experiences an anesthetic response that dissociates the mind from the feelings of being attacked, yet allows the animal to be fully aware of its surroundings. If the predator continues the assault, the victim will not feel the pain so intensely. And, if the predator happens to prefer live prey, the animal can get up once the attacker leaves and scurry off to safety.

I include the freeze response here for two reasons. First, "playing dead" when we feel fear is another way of saying that we have dissociated ourselves from its cause. I first learned of the application of the principle of the freeze response in humans when I was reading Peter Levine's book, *Healing Trauma*. Victims of physical and sexual abuse experience a set of physiological reactions very similar to a jungle animal under attack. Later, they often split their minds off from the reality of what has occurred. They may not be able to retrieve the exact nature of the trauma, but the body holds the memory. Reading about this phenomenon reminded me of a friend who had been forced to play dodge ball at school when she was young. The trauma of being coerced to stand and be hit hard by a ball thrown at her by her classmates stayed with her into adulthood. Any time a ball was involved in a group activity, she could hardly raise her arms to catch it or fend it off. While she would laugh when she told the story of her dodge ball days, the trauma lived on in her body's cells.

In a context of less intensity than severe human trauma, "playing dead" can also occur when we experience fears that I will call "personal-emotional"—fears that exist as a result of our need to protect our fragile egos from attack. Fear of rejection, for example, is something we have all dealt with at one time or another and involves the fear that who we are, what we think, or what we represent will not be good enough to win the love or approval of another person. Often, a fear of rejection is accompanied by the tag-along fear of being alone. We will go to almost any length to protect ourselves from feeling rejected and alone.

One of the ways we accomplish this is to simply "play dead," numb ourselves, immobilize our emotions, stop our connections and communications, anesthetize ourselves with drugs or alcohol, stay there in body, but be "dead" in terms of our hearts and spirits. In such cases, we are basically saying, "I won't risk letting you hurt me." In one of those classic ironies-of-ironies, acting to protect ourselves from the possibility of rejection and loneliness leads us headlong into the path of both.

As you do your practice of the Five Tibetans this week, pay close attention to what your body is telling you. What emotions are rising to the surface? When do they come? In what part of your body are they speaking to you? The physical and meditative practice of the five poses can be a gateway to the release of the held memories of fear that are trapped in your body and in your spirit.

Fear and Grasping

One of my primary goals in writing this book was to give you a safe place to look deeply at behaviors that are holding you back from your greatest calling and your most fulfilling connections. (If it is any comfort, I have spent a good year now being confronted by these same reckonings.) We have identified grasping as a primary agent in the beliefs and actions that limit growth and impact. Grasping can show itself as a need for control when we fear situations and relationships that could potentially require us to confront uncomfortable emotional feelings, such as rejection, disappointment, and failure.

Our compulsion to control our circumstances is a sign that we are deeply attached to the outcomes. We are also equating our safety and well-being with what someone else does or says. Needing to control the outcome is a sign that we do not feel confident enough within ourselves to withstand the personal power of another person. We hang onto our "musts" and "shoulds." We make up rules for ourselves and others. We are convinced that we can leave nothing to anyone else, not even God, a practice that Parker Palmer calls "functional atheism." We believe that if we are not in control of the circumstances, something bad will inevitably occur.

Our fear of losing control will also limit the depth of our connections and communication with the people around us. Intimacy puts us at too great a risk. We cannot afford to delve into knowing the deepest hopes and fears of another human being—not only might it be scary but we also cannot hazard the possibility of a comparison; we certainly cannot risk letting them know us. We keep our gifts, feelings, and thoughts close to the vest. Given that we cannot trust what is in us and around us, we cannot commit ourselves to a life with another human being. Or, maybe we cannot even fathom having a best friend. Any person capable of breaking down our need to control the situation will be seen as a threat. Any situation that might lead to rejection or embarrassment must be avoided. If this pattern persists over a lifetime, we will find our emotional growth stunted and our relationships shallow or nonexistent. Fear can, quite literally, take our lives away.

Bibi, a friend of mine who works with older people at the end of their lives, recently shared with me that she believes our character or individuality is a manifestation of the way we cope with our fears in life. After spending a few seconds being jealous that she thought of it instead of me, I was struck by how true it is.

In her view, we wear a cloak that shields us from our fears. You might also think of it as a mask. As we get older and become more able to lay aside our fears, the cloak gets thinner. We are more able to be our true selves. It is such an amazing picture of how our fears determine how we live our lives. Do we take risks personally or physically? Can we venture out and make the big mistakes? Do we dare to be vulnerable? Can we let ourselves live creatively and expansively? Are we able to hold to our paths and actions regardless of the opinions of others? Can we afford to live intimately with another human being?

Bibi said the picture gave her a new perspective about the people around her. I invite you to spend a little time looking at the fear behind the cloaks that you and the people closest to you wear. In addition to incredible insights, you may also uncover new wells of compassion and forgiveness.

Taking the Learning into Your Practice

I would now like to invite you to explore the learning from this chapter in the midst of doing the Fourth Tibetan. You will be impacting the energy of the second, or sacral, chakra. This chakra is enormously influential: it governs your sense of self and harmonious connection to the world around you. Fear comes from a sense of smallness, mistrust, and judgment. Staying in fear inhibits your creativity and expansiveness and grinds you further into the victim mentality that confusion, resentment, and doubt have started. Fear will not only steal your joy, it will carry away your motivation, your creativity, and your truthfulness with yourself and others.

The Fourth Tibetan is connected to the element of water. We have been designed with an intimate connection to water. Our physical bodies are mostly water. We were born out of water. Water is ingrained in both our evolution and our consciousness. As you lie back to begin the pose, imagine yourself on the surface of a great body of water. Feel the way the water holds you. You are safe. There is no fear. Begin by saying the mantra for the Fourth Tibetan. (*This is water. Opening the belly and sacral chakra. Washing away judgment of myself and others, blame and guilt of myself and others, lack of morality and integrity, smallness and fear. Creating a flow of truth and honor, authenticity, creativity and expansiveness, acceptance and peace.*)

Let the movements of the pose flow like water through your body. As you inhale, you will lift your head and shoulders and then bring up your legs. As you exhale, you will lower your head and shoulders and legs. Feel the rhythm of your breath and of the pose. Imagine yourself like oars in the water, dipping in and moving out. Perform at least three repetitions. (If you are working through the 12-week plan, you may want to perform 11 repetitions.) Focus your attention on the area right below your navel, connecting the doing of the yoga with your sacral chakra.

As you lay back to rest in Corpse Pose, take a moment to feel the blood course within your body. Feel the decelerating beat of your heart. Be with your breath as it slows and resumes its resting rhythm. Visualize now that you are a beautiful leaf traveling along in the eddies and cascades of a small mountain stream, dancing gracefully down toward the river below. See yourself gliding effortlessly in the flow of the stream, moving around this rock and over that obstacle.

As you travel, bring to mind and name the fears that are keeping you small and in judgment of yourself and others. Feel the fears drop away and into the water beneath you. They will stay behind you as you flow ahead. If you are doing the 12-week program, do this visualization each day of this week. If the same fears seem to be returning during the visualization, continue to let them drop to the bottom of the stream. When you notice these fears arise in your daily activities, be aware of the circumstances, of your own perspective, of the feelings that surround them. Record your reactions in your journey journal. By naming your fears and recognizing their work in your life, you will begin to dissolve their power.

Getting Up When You
Have Fallen Down

When your horse throws you, you cannot ride any old horse again; you have to get back on the one that delivered you into the land of fear and doubting. It is not the horse you have to tame; it is the voice inside your head that says you are not able, not enough, not qualified to sit in the saddle and lead a creature of such magnificence.

Fortunately, we had scheduled two Five Tibetans Workshop previews. I knew I had a week to regain my confidence and correct the course. I thought once again about Dr. Brené Brown's confessions in *Daring Greatly*. People—total strangers—had written her hurtful emails after her TED talk took off. They criticized her weight and her fashion sense, and (of course, if you really want to hit a woman where she lives) her dedication as a mother. She had her tears and second thoughts, but she ultimately did a second TED and wrote her book—several books, in fact. The message was not allowed to die simply because the messenger was a human being or because outsiders questioned her ability to deliver it.

As we move into exploring the last nail in the grasping coffin, I want to encourage you to take a moment to reflect on your fear "tells." What messages are you sending out to let others know about your inner, unspoken fears? How are those messages keeping you feeling small and undeserving of the luscious fruits your Creator has prepared for you? Would you be willing to take off the cloak for the sake of enjoying the love and having the impact you were meant to have?

Miserliness

This is earth.
Opening the root chakra.
Covering inferiority and superiority.
Burying arrogance and miserliness and anything
that separates me from others.

I grew up in Claremore, a small town in northeastern Oklahoma. The once-famous cross-country highway, Route 66, runs through the heart of the town; the local museum proudly boasts the original "surrey with a fringe on top" from the Broadway musical *Oklahoma*. Claremore is also home to a memorial dedicated to Will Rogers, the gentleman cowboy. Rogers, who was of Cherokee descent, was among the original political pundits—performing lasso tricks and spinning his folksy political yarns, both on vaudevillian stages and before royalty.

The town was dominated by rural elements when I was growing up. Fields and trees and streams were my playgrounds. When I was a teenager, my friends and I would meet at a small out-of-the-way water reservoir for afternoons of fishing and hanging out. We climbed on the rocks and cast our worm-laden hooks into the cool, green water.

I now know that our fishing hole was the remnant of a strip mine that once produced coal. While Oklahoma is well known as a producer of crude oil and natural gas, I was not aware that coal mining had been a part of the region's economy. It was not until I was teaching a class on energy and the environment that I discovered that eastern Oklahoma had at one time been (and still is in some areas) a rather prolific excavator of the seams of compressed ancient remains of plants that form what we call coal.

Earth is a generous and nurturing Mother. She provides for our needs, continuing to do so even when it puts her at risk. She waves us on as we pollute her waters. She continues to produce as we scrape the forests from her surface. She recycles the air we fill with smog and chemicals. But she has her limits. When we start to dig down into Her core, She gets downright stingy. It becomes a battle of wills: ours against Hers. As a result, mining is a violent process. Dynamite, huge digging machines, and corrosive chemicals are used to take from Her crust what we will to claim for our own gain.

The little reservoir my friends and I visited was a testament to the process of mining. The rocky sides or "high walls" had been created by literally taking the top off the area. In the beginning, the "overburden"—soil and rock that cover the coal seam—are trucked away; toward the end of the process the debris is just left to pile up along the sides. The overall effect is something akin to a moon crater. In the days before regulations for compulsory reclamation, a surface mine that had outlived its usefulness was left to fill with water. Acidic and toxic byproducts resulting from rain water mingling with the mined materials contaminated ground water and were carried down gradient to create hazards for flora, fauna, and humans.

Those open, leftover pits were not only eyesores, they were dangerous, attractive nuisances for kids like me and my friends seeking a place to get away to fish and swim. The waters in an abandoned pit could be 40–70 feet deep, but they had unknown submerged boundaries. Numerous seemingly immortal teens have encountered their mortality diving off rocky highwalls into what turned out to be shallow waters. Children and adults still drown in the deep waters of open mine pits.

Pits of Destruction

The picture of our nurturing and loving Mother Earth ravaged for Her subsurface treasures paints a graphic picture for our consideration of miserliness, the last of the grasping behaviors. Violent blasting of Earth's resources opens gaping wounds that create peril for unsuspecting passersby. Toxic waters form and contaminate land and life downstream.

The mining process produces pits of destruction that can serve as models of what happens to us when our hurts and emotions are left to fester. Have you ever been a pit of destruction? I know I have. Recently I heard someone say something unkind to my sister. I texted her and told her I was sorry the person had been so cruel. She texted back and said, "Wounded people wound people." I had never heard that expression before, but did it ever resonate. I have been that wounded person. I have even described myself as a big, maimed animal swinging its head back and forth and clawing its way through whatever was ahead of it. Have you ever been there—so hurt and shut down that the beast that lurks within was able to come out? Woe to the person who unknowingly steps into that pit at the wrong moment.

Grasping behaviors take you away from connection. They lead you one by one down rickety steps into the pit of personal destruction and isolation. You can feel safe there. It is dark and quiet. No one will bother you. You can find a corner, put your back to the wall, and tell yourself the story that you are better off not needing to deal with other people. No one can hurt you. No one can know you. But one of the consequences of this decision is that while you are shutting out the suffering, you are also closing yourself off to love, joy, and a supportive community. Your gifts are stagnating. Your heart is shriveling. Your confusion, resentment, doubt, and fear create tainted waters that can poison your life and the lives of the people around you.

In this chapter we are going to take an up-close look at "miserliness." The stuff of Old Man Scrooge and the Grinch—and maybe each of us every once in a while. The good news is that we have now reached the bottom of the "grasping" spiral. I invite you to really take on the mining analogy for the next few pages. Suit up to do some exploring of what is below your own surface. When we are done, we will start moving back up the sides of the pit toward our ultimate goal: connection.

The "Mean" in Miserly

Miserliness was my chosen bottom of the grasping realm because it embodies everything I believe takes us away from loving and productive connections with the people around us, namely holding onto what we have and not being willing to share it with anyone. We often associate miserliness with money, but from its Latin origins we know that the word miser referred to an unhappy, wretched, pitiful person. Over time that use of the word faded and was replaced by our current picture of a miser as someone who hoards money. Perhaps a logical extension of the original meaning was that such a person would be intensely unhappy.

Webster's online definition of miserly is "grasping meanness and penuriousness." I had to look up "penuriousness," which means experiencing an oppressive lack of resources or "extreme stinting frugality." To get the full effect of the definition, I will add the British notion of "mean" to the conversation. Mean is one of those words I had to have translated for me by my British friends; in Britain, to be "mean" is to be stingy or tight. That knowledge helped me understand the breadth of Webster's definition of "grasping meanness and penuriousness." The miser, then, is a person who is stingy with himself and others, and will even relegate himself to a life of extreme poverty to hold onto what he has. Based on the origins of the word, we are led to believe that someone who is a miser will endure a life of unhappiness and distress.

Is that not a perfect picture of what happens when someone has gone all the way down to the bottom of the grasping pit? Holding on to confusion and anger and doubt and fear, ending up alone and selfish and impoverished—not destitute, necessarily, but definitely bereft of heart.

The Faces of Miserliness

The concept of miserliness is composed of two important facets: self-abuse and abuse of others. I know that is strong language, and it is exactly what results when we enter the pit of miserliness. A miser is not only mean with others, he is mean with himself as well. He is not only stingy mean, he can also be "not nice" mean. As with resentment, miserliness frequently results from our attempts to protect ourselves—perhaps due to unmet needs, past times of hardship, or a current situation in which we feel our personal resources are being drained and taken for granted. We might feel we have to guard our precious internal resources. Scarcity, whether real or perceived, creates a compulsion to grasp onto possessions or reserves and propels the belief that letting go will result in calamity.

To develop a clearer understanding of the basis for miserliness and what it can bring to—and take away from—our lives, I want to enlist the help of two of literature's most beloved villains, Old Man Scrooge and the Grinch.

Dickens's Scrooge provides us with the quintessential example of a miser, specifically, a financially wealthy old man with no family ties, no friends, and no real creature comforts. He cannot allow himself any ease; he will not provide it for his employee, either. Through the work of the spirit of Christmas Past, we learn that Scrooge himself was often abandoned as a child. In his young adult life, he shunned love in favor of money. He had his regrets, but never worked to correct his missteps. He lived a solitary life and possessed a shriveled heart.

The Grinch in Dr. Seuss's The Grinch Who Stole Christmas lived alone with his little dog Max. Like his mentor Scrooge, we can assume he was very isolated. We are not sure exactly why the Grinch hated Christmas, but we are led to believe he probably had a small heart. What we do know is that he loathed everything about the holiday—presents and feasting and singing. He spent 53 years despising it. The day came when he was no longer content to simply detest the celebration from a distance; he had to take it away from the people who were enjoying it. The Grinch ultimately devised and carried out a plan to dismantle every aspect of Christmas in the village of Who-Ville.

Scrooge and the Grinch give us glimpses of the various aspects of miserliness. Scrooge was stingy with his emotions and finances. He had severed his own love relationship early in life for the pursuit of wealth. He rebuffed his nephew's constant attempts to bring him into the company of others. Scrooge was kind in neither word nor deed. There was no evidence that he had any patience or compassion with anyone in his pre-dream life.

The Grinch was not a financial miser, but we get the sense that he was both personally and spiritually stingy. He could not abide the intimate connection and joy he saw among the folks in Who-Ville. He resented their commitment to each other and to the holiday. The Grinch could turn on the charm when necessary, but he was ruthless and bent on destroying everything he conceived as a source of enjoyment for the Whos.

As you move through this chapter, I want to invite you to look at your own inner Scrooge and Grinch. I suspect that the idea of being miserly impacts people in much the same way as the idea of being resentful does. Who me? After all, I just called Scrooge and the Grinch "villains." Who wants to be thought of as a villain? But while you are here, perhaps you will join me as I explore my own miser. I am already starting to see things pop out of the page at me—situations of late where I have been reluctant or unwilling to give of myself; days, even years, when I have hidden in shame or fear and not shared my gifts with the world; relationships that have suffered because doubt kept me from giving my whole heart. There is probably a little Scrooge or Grinch in all of us. If it helps, ask yourself, "What and where am I holding back?"

How Do You Know Miserliness When You See It?

For most of us, miserliness is not about not sharing our money, but about other treasures we are hoarding, such as time, love, compassion, and forgiveness. I am not saying that every time we say, "No," we are being miserly. Healthy boundaries are a must. I do think we have to examine ourselves when "No" becomes our default. There is nothing wrong with privacy and retreat. But when isolation becomes our norm, then perhaps we have to take a peek into our motives. In retrospect, the times I have hidden out and shut down, I was often hiding from some part of myself that I was either ashamed of or afraid to bring out into the light of day.

As I write this chapter, all my personal alarms are going off and the red-lighted pointers are blinking Time! Time! Time! I tried my best to ignore the signals, but is it possible that I am miserly with my time? I have lived with moderate resources for so long I am fairly adept at believing that money comes in and goes out and I can share it without hesitation. But time? That is another issue.

Right now, with a book deadline, and a business to start, and a class to teach—let me just say, woe to the one who steps into that mix wanting to claim some of my time for a reason I might deem insignificant! I hunker down over time like Scrooge over the money box and guard it at all costs. I sit and write. Get up and eat. Sit back down and write. Take a walk. Sit down and write. I am not seeking any outlets. I am rarely offering to make time for other things. In my mind, I defend this behavior by saying that I have a contract to meet and a job to do. That is all true, but how am I going about it? Like it or not, I am aware that disturbing patterns are developing.

Beware the Miser's Cave

Let me analyze the "tells" of miserliness from my own confession. First, there is physical withdrawal. When you step near my work cave, I am not generous. I do not look up and smile and exude warmth. I will literally withdraw my body. I will resist making eye contact because I do not want you to know I have seen you. In my mind, I am thinking that if I did not see you, you won't see me either, and you will go away and I can continue what I am doing.

Second, my short temper and impatience will surface. If you are less than perceptive and step into the cave, even though I am sending all my "best" signals, chances are I will not be nice. I might be exasperated. I will snarl a bit. The beast will be making its way into the light of day.

Third, resentment steps in. If you do persist, and I do give you whatever you are seeking, I will assuredly do it with a reluctance and ill will. I will be well into the pit by now. I will not be able to see your need; I will be fully focused on my perceived personal injury.

Ouch. This is a painful analysis. Let me go even farther into this fetid muck with one final admission: I will resort to blame and judgment. I will be thinking the whole time that it is YOU who is being disrespectful and unappreciative. After all, can you not see that I am busy doing important work here? What is it that you need to have done that is more important than what I have to do?

Am I miserly with my time? Have I been grasping? Yes, I am hanging onto the precious moments of my time. Have I been stingy? Yes, I have been unwilling to share my time with you. Have I withheld myself and my gifts from you? And have I engineered the situation so that any good that might have come to me has been extinguished? Yes. There I am in the dictionary, right under "grasping meanness and penuriousness."

It is quite horrifying to see it all so plainly. As with all of our grasping behaviors, miserliness appears in the least of circumstances, as well as the moments of greatest importance. Perhaps we are better able to admit to and explore miserliness in those lesser instances.

I invite you to take a few moments to consider the four "tells" from my self-analysis: physical withdrawal, impatience, resentment, and blame and judgment. How do these resonate with your own encounters with miserliness? If need be, start thinking about another person you consider to be miserly. What is she withholding? Love? Affection? Money? Time? Kindness? Communication? Compassion? Forgiveness? How do you know?

Once you have a picture of what miserliness looks like in another, let the pointer finger begin to turn inward to yourself. Close your eyes and consider areas where miserliness might creep into your daily interactions with others. Be gentle. I would not want for you the pummeling I gave myself when I was writing this chapter. We are on an expedition into the pit. This is our laboratory. Be as thorough and as objective as you can be.

The good news is that we all do it; you are not alone. We all have moments when we cannot find it within ourselves to give freely from open and generous hearts—when out of confusion or hurt or doubt or fear, we step into the pit of selfishness and smallness. My perspective on it is that you simply stay aware. Keep looking within when you feel the beast coming out. You may not catch it in that moment. Or the next. Or the next. But your mindfulness will have its perfect result in time.

Before we move on, I invite you to look into one more corner. Are there areas where you are miserly in your interactions with yourself? Do you nurture yourself? Forgive yourself? Love yourself? Do you have compassion for yourself? Generally speaking, if you cannot be generous with yourself, you cannot be truly charitable with anyone else either. The times when I am shut down and cannot give freely to others, I am inevitably in a situation where for one reason or another, I am not giving to myself, either. I am working too many hours. I am driven by some purpose or another. I am running on empty and feel I have nothing in my tank to offer someone else. If you do not take anything else away from this discussion of miserliness, please look into how you are caring for yourself. Weary, lonely, and limping, you will create a perfect breeding ground for a retreat into the pit of miserliness.

Taking Miserliness into Your Practice

We withhold from ourselves and others for many reasons. At times, it is generated from an unconscious belief that we are not worthy of attention or graciousness. Sometimes we are living with guilt and regrets that we are unable to resolve. More than likely, however, miserliness is spawned by a deep-seated belief that the world is not a safe and nurturing place.

The Fifth Tibetan opens the root (first) chakra. When you find yourself approaching a miserly moment, you may want to visualize that deep dark expanse of the seat of your primal support and foundation. It is the gateway to the feminine in you, the place of your birth. Visualizing roots going down into Mother Earth from your root chakra will help you gain a clearer and stronger connection to the nature of this chakra. When the root chakra is balanced, you are secure and generous. You are confident that you can afford to give and receive material possessions, as well as love and affection. You are big in heart and deed. When the first chakra is not in balance, however, distrust of the world around you and a sense of scarcity and lack can develop. It is from these roots that miserliness grows, creating a compulsion to hold onto what you have—to focus on material goods, to never feel that you have (or are) enough.

I want to take a moment to acknowledge something here. I know that many of you who read this book have experienced sexual and/or physical abuse in your lifetime. It is so prevalent in the culture that few of us have escaped its reality. When I suggest that you focus on the earth being a "safe" place, I do not mean to insinuate that you have never encountered danger or a lack of personal safety. I am proposing that you connect to the knowing that you are held by the goodness and generosity of the earth beneath you.

If, in fact, you have experienced abuse, it is very likely that your root chakra is in need of loving healing work. You may find yourself experiencing strong emotions in this chapter. I encourage you to remain curious. Always go gently into your contemplations. Awareness will make room for healing over time. If your memories and emotions begin to overtake you, you may want to seek the help of a counselor or healer who can hold your words and your wounds as you move through the process.

This seems a good time to stop and go through a few repetitions of the Fifth Tibetan. I confessed earlier that it is my favorite pose. I enjoy feeling my body work with the fluidity of the movements and the breath. As you perform the pose now, focus your awareness on your body in the beginning of the pose. Your hips are up in the air and your head is tucked between your arms. Physically, you are vulnerable to attack. Geographically, you have distanced yourself from the earth. You have both moved away from the source of your nurture and retreated into your own little world. As you move back down into the "sag," feel your renewed connection with the ground beneath you. Feel the power in your body. Notice the sense of grounding. You are confident and competent. You are not a victim of your past, or of your fears and doubts. If possible, perform at least three repetitions of the Fifth Tibetan at this time.

Explore the way the pose impacts your sense of connection to the nurture and provision of the earth.

As you move into Child's Pose to rest, cuddle down next to Mother Earth. Be willing to let go of the secret hurts that lie beneath your surface. The physical exertion of 21 repetitions of the Fifth Tibetan frequently sets me up for a release of emotion in the rest pose. As always, when emotions come, please do not hinder them: their purpose is to cleanse old wounds and clear the decks to make room for your next big leap in life. Just imagine that you are being held in a space of unconditional love and provision. Allow yourself to indulge in a moment of absolute safety. If you desire, visualize a crystal pyramid forming around you, creating a powerful and beautiful barrier between you and any energy or person not contributing to your highest good. Feel the cool glassy surface next to your forehead. Visualize the apex above you refracting all the colors of the rainbow. See yourself in the midst of all that beauty and light. Breathe.

Final Thoughts

The realization that I hoard time was overwhelming to me. I had an inkling that it might be true, but I had no idea of the extent of it until I allowed myself to look at it straight on. In the realm of money, I always say, "Money comes in and money goes out. It is like breathing. Don't hold your breath." Granted, money is slightly different from time, but I believe the principle is similar no matter the resource we are considering. What you hang onto cannot multiply. Time, money, gifts, love, forgiveness, communication, and compassion all expand as they are given. The more tightly we hold onto them, the less abundant they become and the more destitute of spirit we become.

That is, in essence, the story on miserliness. If we hold onto ourselves, our talents, or our resources, we stand to lose everything. It is only when we give of ourselves and what has been graced to us that we can create the security and abundance we desire.

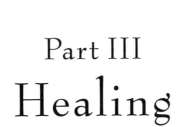

Part III
Healing

Change is Inevitable,
Therefore, It Is Possible

I *was walking along the sidewalk in an upper middle-class neighborhood in central North Carolina. It was mid-April. Spring had sprung. The cherry trees were in blossom. The redbud trees were adorned with their tight reddish/purple blooms. Tulips and daffodils rose above the thick dark green rye grass lawns and monkey grass borders. The sky overhead was a clear blue—no clouds in sight. The breeze was gentle, and as usual, the humidity was on the rise.*

I saw them as I crested the hill coming across an intersection where the main road branched off into a cul-de-sac. She was dressed casually: three-quarter-length pants and a purple lightweight long-sleeved shirt; he was outfitted for outdoor work in the sun and heat: short-sleeved green shirt, khaki work pants, heavy gloves. They stood there talking. As I approached, I heard her say to him that she hoped he had a good weekend. He replied that he would be praying for her. She turned and went back into her upper-middle-class, two-story house; he went back to edging the sidewalk on the side nearest the street.

At first glance, you would not think this to be anything other than two people talking. He was the "yard man"; she was the "lady of the house." It was so normal. And yet, it was a scene that would have created a scandal (perhaps worse) a mere 50 years ago—this woman of color talking to a white man out in plain sight in a small town in North Carolina.

As I approached the two, I began to think about all that had happened both in our country as a whole and in the South to create this opportunity for two people to stand on the sidewalk and have a chat. We take it for granted now. Most of us cannot even imagine it any other way.

Some months back, I wrote in my journal, "Change is inevitable, therefore, it is possible." Reading You Are Here *drove that point home to me over and over again. Change is inevitable. And only because change is inevitable do we enjoy the world as we know it. Seeds sprout to become flowers and trees. Flowers die back to make way for the plump seeds forming within the ovary. Seasons give way to one another. Lakes ice over and thaw. We are totally dependent on the reality that everything changes. And, because change is an ever-occurring event, it is possible. The world can change. Societies can change. People can change.*

One day, after years of racial tension and conflict, a black woman can stand on a street in the Deep South and talk openly with her white yard man.

We can change. Our hearts can change. I can change.

CHAPTER 9

Awareness

This is light.
Opening the Third Eye.
Lighting the way for wisdom and insight,
clarity and perspective, reality and awareness,
acceptance, and peace.

It sat on the edge of the North Sea, balanced on the final inches of a dune that gave way abruptly onto the shingle and beach below. Like a bull's eye at the end of the world, the grand labyrinth of pebbles and rocks looked out into the endless waters that terminated hundreds of miles away in the Arctic Circle. It was a spiraling structure created over time by the ones who came to seek peace and spiritual enlightenment in the place known as Findhorn.

The first time I walked the labyrinth, I was awestruck by the views of the North Sea and dunes and windmills and sky. I could sense the hearts and intentions of the many people who had walked the labyrinth for their varied reasons. Occasionally, a rock with a message or even a branded piece of wood provided a clue as to the needs and visions of those who had followed the path. On one visit, I found an oval stone with the word SECURITY painted on it placed on the low wall of rocks leading to the center. Another time, I noticed a small stuffed gray elephant planted among the rocks and shells and feathers that formed the stony center stage of the labyrinth. Who placed them there? For what purpose? Much like the walk of the labyrinth, each person had to make up her own meanings for the artifacts left behind by predecessors.

When I returned to enjoy a second late fall in Scotland, I immediately made my way over the dunes and down to the labyrinth. Despite its location in the path of strong winds and rains, little had changed in the 10 months since I had first walked the labyrinth's winding paths. The most notable addition was a large, domed pile of sand that had been caught up in a bunch of dune grass, a growth that straddled one of the lines of rocks in the outer ring. My first impression was that it resembled a hairy mole on an old woman's face. It seemed appropriate somehow, adding wisdom and gentleness, reminding me of the inevitability of aging and change.

The dunes along the ocean are public. No one owns the space. The labyrinth is on the leg of the Moray Coastal Trail that runs between Findhorn Village and the little royal burg of Burghead. Burghead is known for its ability to attract the bottlenose dolphins that swim about in the cold waters of this part of the North Sea. Many people pass the labyrinth each day—Findhorn seekers, families, dog walkers, horses with riders. As a result, the odd obstacle forced me to wait or alter my course as I took the journey to the labyrinth's center. Dogs and children would scurry past in front of me, and I frequently had to skirt large piles of manure left by a rider's steed. Generally, I would laugh or sidestep and move on.

My equanimity met its match one clear, windy November morning. I was about halfway around the path when a middle-aged woman and her son came over a nearby dune and seemed to make their way toward the labyrinth. They hovered near the entrance to the path, talking loudly enough to be heard over the wind and surf. The son proceeded to descend the steep sandy cliff onto the levy made of shingles (stones) and on down the beach to the water.

The woman stood for a moment and then walked over the rocks and paths of the labyrinth, moving across its expanse from one side to the other along the fragile edge that lay at the end of the dune. She stopped in the space of the far path, watching her son as he walked on the beach below. I continued my journey along the labyrinth, coming very close to the woman on one of my journeys round. After a few minutes, the mother called out to her son. He came up from the beach, joined her, and they made their way back the way they had come in.

Meanwhile, back in the maybe-now-not-so-meditative aura of the labyrinth, I was trying to focus on understanding rather than criticizing what for all the world looked to me like a blatant disregard and lack of respect for a place dedicated to silence and meditation. Well, perhaps there was just a smidge of criticism. What *were* they thinking? Seeing me going round and round and back and forth, was it not obvious to them that this place was not just another stretch of sand among the dunes?

Trying to make sense of other people's behavior can be a confusing process. I struggled to see the labyrinth through their eyes. They came for a peek at the sea. It just so happened that this big rock-strewn structure took up a prime piece of real estate between them and the beach. I still could not grasp it, though. The woman stood right on top of the labyrinth. She walked over it. She stepped on the rocks and stood in one of the paths. If it had been me... Soon, I was off on one of those internal spins where I was giving her a piece of my mind. (Perhaps it is worth mentioning at this point that when you attempt to give someone a piece of your mind, you invariably forfeit your *peace* of mind, as we shall see here.)

Conflicting Values

Eventually, a bit of mindfulness crept in, and I got hold of the round-and-round-we-go monologue. It was time to change course for a minute. If it had been me, I reasoned, I would have known it was a labyrinth. I would have understood that people in it were in a state of meditation or personal contemplation. I would have moved down the sand a bit to find a place to talk and stand that would not have interfered with the purpose of the labyrinth.

At this point, the light dawned. I would do all those things because I value the labyrinth and what it represents. I value it as a tool for spiritual reflection. I value the time someone put in to set it up. It has value to me, personally. I had held the labyrinth in my memory for a year and could not wait to walk it when I came back to Findhorn. The wants and needs of the woman and her son were different from mine. I wanted to engage in spiritual practice; they wanted to stand by the sea. I wanted silence; they needed to communicate. As it turned out, our wants and needs clashed.

We find ourselves among people with incongruent values all the time. They eat meat; we do not. We go to church; they do not. Their kids watch television; ours do not. The list is endless. Each and every item on our list represents not only what we value but also points to where we put our attention, the insights we have been given, and our perception of the world. Each value is a composite of the mental, emotional, and spiritual constructions we have made over the course of our lives.

So I felt like I had figured it out. The lesson was about valuing, and how valuing impacts the way we look at the things other people are doing; therefore, I could just chalk up the interruption to a mismatch of what I and they valued. Fine. Yes, but I'm sorry... Really? Could they not see that someone was in the process of walking the labyrinth? Kids and dogs. I get that. Exuberant children and frolicking canines are generally unaware of their impact on others unless forced to in some way. I just assume that adults have some sort of built-in other-people's-space-awareness.

At that juncture, the lesson seemed to be shifting focus to a connection between valuing and awareness. That sent me into a round of Twenty Questions. Can you really be aware of something that you do not value? Are we basically blind to the things we do not value? Do our different value systems make it difficult to see something that is literally right in front of our noses? How often do I walk on or over something important to another person, oblivious to its value for them because it has no value for me?

I could see myself heading into one of those tangles of terminology and semantics—awareness, valuing, some of both. Under all that ruminating, however, still lay the real issue I needed to resolve. How do I hold my center when someone or something important to me is threatened? How can I transform criticism and confusion regarding the actions of other people into insight and awareness? What can I do when I get in that spin of what-I-would-do-if-it-were-me and how-can-they-be-so-oblivious?

As I recently reread my journal entry about the incident, I realized that there was more to it than a conflict between their values and mine or their lack of awareness. I was convinced I was missing an important piece, one that might help me better sort things out on those occasions when I am tempted to react negatively when the needs and values of others encroach on my space. Reluctantly, I knew it was time to turn the telescope around and make me the star for a moment. I had focused on "them" for long enough. Resolution was not going to happen until I took a closer look at my own role in this drama at the labyrinth.

Awareness Matters

From a spiritual perspective, awareness is the ability to observe all that is in and around us without being carried off by any stories our minds try to tell us. In the *Power of Now*, Eckhart Tolle suggests that to accomplish this being-with-all-that-is-and-remaining-detached-from-it, we must invoke the process of "watching the thinker." To accomplish that, you let the mind run like a movie and sit back and observe the show. You do not judge the content, or yourself, or others.

The spiritual seat for this kind of removed yet actively involved awareness is the Third Eye chakra. As you learned earlier, the First Tibetan focuses on opening the Third Eye, considered by many ancient traditions to be the seat of insight and awareness. It is the portal into seeing the Divine in ourselves and others, serving as a control panel for our spiritual, emotional, mental, and physical being. When functioning optimally, this chakra shines a powerful light on our lives and our thoughts, thus allowing us the gift of perspective. We can be with the past and the present and the future and see the Divine handiwork in all of it. We can be in the here-and-now, aware and centered.

When we are able to know our truth and to believe that everything is happening for some purpose, we can be in a state of peaceful awareness. People or things that move into and out of our space are not allowed to throw us off our center. All that sounds very nice and easy ... on paper. In the day-to-day world, however, reality, clarity, and awareness can be difficult to work with. That hurt that just came into your life—it is there for a perfect reason. The relationship that just failed—its ending is in your best interest. The abuse from your childhood—simply fodder for the work you are meant to do in the world.

I do not always arrive at those perspectives so easily. How am I to simply ignore people and events around me that bring pain and chaos into my life just because they might be part of some bigger plan that I cannot see at the time? A rather unfortunate situation gave me the opportunity to explore this process further. I had a friend who had two experiences with ovarian cancer in four years. She had gone into the hospital the day after Christmas at the time I was writing this book and seemed to be rapidly deteriorating. At the time, I was in France staying with a friend so that I could concentrate on my writing. Realizing that I might need to fly back to the States to be with her, I immediately went into a spin of resistance and reticence—not because I did not want to be with my friend, but because I was sure that, as my finances were literally at their end, I would not be able to get back to France. If I did not get back to France, where would I live and how would I get the book finished? As I was once again out in the world without a home base, that created fear and doubt and apprehension about my circumstances. And that was mixed not so nicely with my guilt, as my friend was very likely facing the end of her life.

I felt the spin coming. There was a lot going on around me and in me. I practiced cuddling my pain and angst close and letting all the feelings surface, being fully with what was arising rather than judging it or running away. Given full permission, the feelings came: resistance, fear, anger. Tears followed. I sat with it all in meditation. I do not want to run away from the parts of me that create resistance and confusion. I want to look into them further. This is harder than it sounds, especially when what I am thinking or feeling puts me in a dim light (*I am not supposed to want* that *or think* that *or feel* that. *What is wrong with me?*). But if I don't take those things out and look at them, they will plague me from the sidelines and likely blindside me later. When I shine the light on my emotions and shadows, I can see *me* better.

I have a favorite picture of my grandson taken when he was a toddler. We were playing with a cardboard carton. He was down on his hands and knees with his head stuck in the box. That is a fairly vulnerable position to be in—your head in a dark space and your backside sticking out. That sums up how it feels when I am faced with coming to grips with my emotions and thoughts in the midst of reacting to and resisting something. I feel vulnerable. Some old wound is rising, and I become afraid that it will carry me off.

In this case, my story (*I will not be able to get back to France where I can stay and write my book*) was accompanied by an assumption (*I have no other options*). The assumption not the story was the culprit. Our stories—our constructions of reality in our world—are natural emanations from our thought life, our sense-making machinery. The stories come and go and cause little harm if we can avoid attaching to them or insisting they become international best-sellers. Those cheeky assumptions, on the other hand, can be trickier. They come from a deeper place, from our beliefs about ourselves and the world around us. So my story was undergirded by an assumption that was actually a manifestation of a belief. In this case, the belief was likely, "I am a prisoner to the limited money in my bank account."

This seemed like a good place to invoke one of the four key questions from Byron Katie's "The Work": Is it true? Is it true that my current bank account is the only source of a ticket to/from the States? Is it true that once I leave France, I will not be able to come back? Looking in again from this vantage point, I could see that, no, it was not true. I had other options. Flying to the States to be with my friend was not a commitment to let go of what I had come to France to accomplish. If my belief is not true, then what is true, and how do I keep myself open to the possibilities rather than shutting down as a result of my assumptions?

Awareness is a slippery slope. Being able to observe all that is around us without being taken in by the stories and emotions helps us remain present and at peace. But being with all those stories and emotions, even at a distance, can be a painful work. In order to be aware of ourselves, we have to be willing to dive into our reality. In this case, I needed to be aware of my assumptions and the underlying beliefs. That awareness had to come without judgment or labels. If I started judging my feelings, I would want to run away from them. If I ran away, there was no chance I would be able to do the work I needed to do to stay in the present moment and be with what was happening.

I want to say straight out, on behalf of all of us who do this, it is courageous work. If it were easy, everyone would be doing it. We know for a fact that our friends and family are not always willing to take on their feelings and chase them to their end points. It is essential that when you are in this work, you lavish yourself with gentleness and compassion. Beating yourself up over your reality will not solve the current dilemma and it will discourage you from looking in next time. In this case, once I acknowledged my resistance to what seemed to be coming and was honest about my fears and feelings, I was freer to see that I could do all the things that were important to me rather than feel trapped by the illusion that first popped up.

Steps to Awareness

The process I took away for my self-awareness exploration was fairly simple. First, when the stories come, listen to the language. Words like "never" and "must" and "should" and "always" are great signals that the story is likely not true and needs further examination.

Next, be willing to shine a light on the assumptions. Avoid the urge to run away and hide from your own reality. Take out a big "head torch," as my British friends call it, and go in fearlessly. Look in all the corners of the box. Drag all of those assumptions out in the open so that you can get a big picture view of what is going on in your head.

Finally, look into the beliefs that are hiding under the assumptions. If looking into your assumptions is dirty work, going down into your beliefs can be like crawling through a manhole cover into the sewer below. This is the seat of your values. It is also the place where your gremlins hide. So be courageous and curious. Hold your nose if you need to, but do not back away until you have done a complete inventory. What do you believe about yourself? What do you believe about others? How are those beliefs limiting you?

Going into Your Practice of the First Tibetan

My goal in situations like the drama at the labyrinth and the dilemma about going stateside is to become centered and calm. I know that once I have achieved that, I will be much more able to make decisions that are aligned with my values. That process requires a commitment to transform whatever emotions may be overtaking me into something I can be with more productively. In the situations I described here, I wanted to transform my confusion or irritation or panic or fear into a perspective that would allow me to consider and be with my feelings but not carried away by them.

I have found the First Tibetan to be a good teacher in this process. As noted in our earlier discussion of the pheasant, the spins of the First Tibetan are apt models of who we become when we are off balance, panicky, or afraid—dizzy, going nowhere. If you are following along with the 12-week program, you have now had several weeks of experience doing this yoga and are well aware of the way it impacts your body. Have you tried doing it when you are confused or panicked?

If you are in a safe place, this would be a good time to perform a few repetitions of the First Tibetan. Today, I am going to invite you to explore ways to see transformation in the midst of the spins. In other words, how could this exercise model the process of transforming confusion or fear into awareness and perspective?

I discovered the answer for myself by accident the day after I quite strongly told a friend that I did not receive any insights doing the yogas, and instead found the lessons in the rest positions. Well, never say never. The next morning, as I performed the First Tibetan, I received an insight into the events at the labyrinth at Findhorn that had been bothering me. It happened in the following way.

I was spinning in the First Tibetan, and after each spin made a visual connection with the light of my candle, which served as my point of reference. By looking at the candle flame, I could regain my balance and center myself before the next spin. I also use my reference point as a point of transformation. The short time that I focused on the candle provided a split second of concentrated awareness before the next rotation began. When my eyes focused on the reference point, the whirling view of whatever was going around me as I spun was transformed into one perfectly clear and still picture. That is what I am seeking from awareness—a way to bring about a clear picture of the situation in the middle of fuzzy and upsetting circumstances.

Initially, as I spun on this morning, I considered where I fly when panic and confusion overtake me. Then the question changed to: *Where do I look when I encounter obstacles or irritations? What is my reference point when I need to "stop the spin" and ground myself?*

I thought back to that day on the labyrinth and its spectacular beauty. I had the North Sea in front of me and the soothing sound of the waves breaking on the beach in my ears. I was in the midst of my walking meditation on the labyrinth's paths. What did I choose to focus on? The two people who came over the dunes and into my field of view. I put my awareness on the interruption rather than the joy of my practice, on the actions of others rather than my own pursuit. In the end, I reached the center of the labyrinth but did not transform my thoughts and attitudes on the way.

I wish I could continue to attribute the story of the woman and her son at the labyrinth to their lack of awareness or our conflicting values. It seems, however, that the real issue was mine; the fact is that I lost *my* sense of awareness and allowed their actions to come into my space and, for even a short amount of time, disrupt my spiritual practice and goals. Awareness is meant to give me the ability to be with what is happening in my space, even, and especially when, there are things that are prone to take me off my center and distract me from the work I am meant to be doing in the world. In the end, I had to acknowledge that the incident at the seaside that day had nothing to do with anyone else. It was about me. I was the one who allowed the disruption of my walk along the labyrinth. I was the one who left my focused pursuit of the path and let the actions of others ooze in and destroy the peace that had been created. My own lack of awareness was the cause of my unsettling.

Where do you look when the words or actions of others threaten to take you off your focus? Seeking to find the blame in "them" will likely increase the spin and invariably cause a wobble. You have to catch yourself. Find a "reference point," a place for your focus that will bring you back to balance and center. In many cases, that focal point will be your own story, complete with its assumptions, beliefs, and emotions. That can be a gift. Excavating the good stuff and clearing out the garbage can have transformative effects on the present situation, as well as on events in the future.

You might consider practicing the First Tibetan yoga when situations like this arise. Do a single, purposeful spin. Take in your reference point. What do you see? What do you feel? Where is the resistance? What is the emotion? Do another spin. Again, set your eyes on the transformation point. Go inside and see if you can spot the source of your interior wobbles. You might do a couple of spins, or many. It will depend on how deeply buried the feelings are being held.

After you complete the spins, lie down and rest in Child's Pose. It may take a few seconds for the feeling of the spin to dissipate. Breathe deeply. Let the thoughts go. Be with any emotions that arise. Cradle them close to your heart. Scan your body for any pains or aches that are asking to be acknowledged. An achy knee? A stiff shoulder? A headache brewing? These flags are meant to draw your attention in toward your own center. They are speaking to you. Take a moment to listen carefully. I find that specifically focusing my attention on the ache and verbally acknowledging the discomfort often causes the soreness to dissipate.

Awareness starts in your own space. Insight and clarity are possible when you have the courage to look deeply at what is in and around you—and the wisdom to hold it lightly. Before you arise from the rest pose today, take a moment to acknowledge your own courage and your dedication to the process of deep looking and awareness.

CHAPTER 10

Vulnerability

This is air.
Opening the heart chakra.
Creating space for love and compassion,
for forgiveness and vulnerability,
and for acceptance and peace.

I had accepted a spring semester job as an extra-hire naturalist at Walker Creek Ranch in Marin County, California. In my time there, I learned about the fauna and flora of the area, things such as newts and miner's lettuce. Answering to the camp name of "Flame," I took children on hikes and facilitated games and activities in places dubbed Jack Rabbit Flats and Turkey Vulture Canyon. I dunked my head in Turtle Pond to model the Polar Bear Club initiation process and ate apples—cores, seeds, and all—to demonstrate that all parts are edible. I kissed banana slugs and stuffed the leaves of the California bay laurel (*Umbellularia californica*) into my nostrils. It was a complete experience.

While I enthusiastically accepted all the required activities and challenges, I had a secret, one that was going to have to come out sooner or later: I was absolutely snake phobic, for those of us old enough to remember, about as ophidiophobic as Harrison Ford's Indiana Jones in *Raiders of the Lost Ark*. I could remain calm enough to take the group quietly around the odd four-foot gopher snake lying across the trail. I would check the head shape first, of course, as gopher snakes can be mistaken for rattlesnakes, and vice versa. The two snakes have similar markings and, although I am not certain what evolutionary process made it possible, the harmless gopher snake is able to emulate the sound of its poisonous counterpart by pointing its tail into the leaves and shaking it to make a rattling sound.

The week of reckoning came near the end of April, when the spring rains had turned the hills to green and swelled the creeks and pond so that the California newts were easy to locate and bring out of the water for inspection, their orange bellies warning predators that they were extremely poisonous. You can kiss or lick a banana slug; you absolutely do not kiss an orange-bellied newt.

I was teaching a group of sixth-graders from the Bay Area that week, a pleasant mix of rambunctious 11-year-old boys and "I don't want to get my shoes dirty" girls. (By the end of the week, the girls were more than willing to dive head first into the mud on the trail.) We were assigned to the Lab as a place to start our days and gather before our night hike. The Lab was a large room, not as cozy as some of the spaces, but it was adjacent to the museum that held the refurbished carcasses of a variety of local creatures, as well as bones, rocks, and "ancient" artifacts. The Lab also had a well-known inhabitant: a three-foot-long boa named Shy.

The moment the kids in my group laid eyes on the large glass terrarium housing Shy, they started talking about getting her out and holding her. I had been in that space before and had ducked the bullet because Shy had been molting (and could be irritable and "bitey" so no holding was allowed), but I knew from the first day of this week that things were going to play out differently this time. My trail group would force me to remove Shy and get to know her up close and personal. I was going to have to reach into the cage, put my hands on her, and bring her out. I courageously (perhaps stupidly) told them we would take her out of her house before we went on our night hike.

When I went to the naturalists' area for the afternoon meeting, I asked questions about how best to get the snake out, what to be careful for, and so on, and some of the more experienced naturalists gave me information and pointers. I did not let on that I was uncomfortable about it, because I was not actually "uncomfortable"; I was terrified. I was hoping, in fact, that the snake might mysteriously disappear overnight ... given that there were a couple of nights left, it could still happen.

Our night hike was scheduled for Wednesday. We had been in the room with Shy for two days now, and anticipation was rising. I started the lesson with night hike basics: how our eyes see at night; *diurnal,* nocturnal, and crepuscular animals; and the star formations that we might see. We discussed how snakes fit into the day/night activity timeline and a little about the place Shy would have lived in the wild. Finally, the moment I had been dreading arrived: I would need to get the snake out of the glass enclosure, hold her, and pass her around the class.

The night hike itself brought its own tension. Many of the children who come to Walker Creek Ranch live in cities along the East Bay, where walking alone in the dark is not advisable. They carry that fear into walking alone in the stillness and safety of the country as well. I stood at the front of the room and said, "Tonight we will be taking a night hike. I have heard that some of you are nervous about it. I want to share something that I am nervous about." I went on to tell them that I was afraid of snakes and had never touched or handled a snake.

I did not receive a lot of criticism about my confession, as several of the students were more afraid of the snake than I was—yes, hard to imagine. I then asked if anyone had experience with snakes. One of the boys, Sam, said he had a boa at his father's house. He knew how to hold the snake and agreed to help me.

Sam was a quiet, well-mannered 11-year-old boy. His large dark eyes and thick hair reflected his Latin American descent. He was smaller than most of the boys in the group. He came over to the cage, and we stood looking at it together, our backs to the other students. He helped me get the lid off the top.

I stepped back and took a deep breath. I said, "I think I am going to need some moral support," and held out my left hand, palm up. He looked up at me and without hesitating placed his pudgy sixth-grade boy-hand in mine. He kept holding it while he instructed me about how to lift Shy out of the enclosure and the proper way to hold her. Sam only let go of me when I asked if he wanted to take the snake to show the class.

I watched as Sam held the boa to his body, as a mother might cuddle a young baby, and carried Shy to the area where his peers were sitting. He stood in front of the class with the boa's head in one hand and its tail wrapping around his other arm. The class "oooohed" and "aaahhhed" and "eewed." At that point, I was off the hook. Shy was in experienced hands. It turned out that one of our cabin leaders also had a boa at home and helped Sam pass the snake around the room to allow other students to hold her. All I had to do at this point was breathe and admire this young man, who stood tall and fearless with the snake in his gentle grasp.

Vulnerability

I knew the story of Sam and the boa would be in this book. I treasured it and kept it alive in my memory for more than two years. It was a magical moment of intimacy and compassion. I still get tears in my eyes when I remember holding out my hand and seeing Sam reach out and take it. He had so many options. He was an 11-year-old boy, yet he stepped up in that moment like a wise old sage who knew what was at stake and was not willing to force me to do my work alone.

As we continue with our exploration of the healing behaviors, we will be taking a look at vulnerability. Unlike resentment, which grows from the ill winds of bitterness, anger, and jealousy, vulnerability flourishes in the warm breezes of love, compassion, and forgiveness. Our ability to be vulnerable will dictate the life we live, the relationships we have, and the degree to which we manifest our dreams. It is a measure of both our willingness to fail and our willingness to allow others to fail. The essence of vulnerability reaches down into our very belief about our humanity. We are fallible; our friends are fallible. We hurt people; people hurt us. As a result, we cannot thrive without love and compassion for ourselves and others.

The word "vulnerable" has its root in a Latin word meaning "to wound." We are vulnerable when we are prone to physical or emotional harm. The essence, then, of being vulnerable is to be wound-able. As I was doing the research for this book, I came across a TED talk by Dr. Brené Brown. Watching her talks on vulnerability and shame led me to read her book *Daring Greatly,* where she defines vulnerability as "uncertainty, risk, and emotional exposure" (p. 41). Wow! That more or less covers every minute of every day of your life. It is precisely because of vulnerability's omnipresence that the degree to which you are able to stand in your vulnerability, to remain in the midst of "uncertainty, risk, and emotional exposure," will determine the course of your life.

Vulnerability is Being and Doing

As I have pondered the concept of vulnerability, I have determined that it has two primary faces. First, there is the vulnerability we experience as a result of something people can find to criticize about us: our clothes, our skin color, our acne, our weight, our inability to play baseball or dance, our fear of snakes. The list is endless. We are constantly going to have the opportunity to fail to live up to someone's standards in some way. We do not actually have to do anything wrong to receive this criticism. This is a vulnerability of being, not doing. It comes as a result of people seeing us as different or undesirable in some way. This is the nightmare of being an adolescent. Who you are is the very thing that puts you at risk. You want to "be in" and know that there is no way you can please everyone in every way. Some of us stop attempting to fit in about then. Some of us spend the rest of our lives trying to get it right—to become what will please everyone around us. This aspect of vulnerability ultimately dictates the degree to which we can be our authentic selves.

The second face of vulnerability is about doing. We made a mess, failed, or wounded someone. We actually did something to bring on the risk. We wet our pants at school. We failed an exam. We struck out in the bottom of the ninth inning with the bases loaded. We said something to hurt someone. We broke our grandmother's priceless antique urn. We might feel shame or guilt or fear and never be able to make the thing right, take the words back, or fix it. We retreat, stop trying, quit the team, or walk out of the relationship. To work our way back from these types of episodes, we have to master the art of recovery. The most important aspects of that process are compassion and forgiveness—in this case, for yourself.

I recently got a refresher course in self-forgiveness and compassion. I had spent the summer out of the country. When I got back to the States, I found myself unable to come to the computer to work on the book; instead, I kept myself occupied, cleaned the house, graded papers. The first day it seemed reasonable, as I was making a transition from travel. The second day, I was aware that it might be more than jet lag. By the third day, I had to admit I was avoiding the reality of thinking about the book.

I had spent the summer in a work situation that had drained me and rocked me off my center; I was never able to truly find my feet. Not only did I let myself get unbalanced but I also put angry words and negative energy into the situation around me. I had fallen into every grasp-oriented trap imaginable—resentment, jealously, doubt, and miserliness—and had left the place feeling a great deal of shame. After all, I was writing a book about healing from such things. What good were my words if I could not even pull it off for myself?

In fact, reading what I had already written left me feeling more shame. The pheasant? I had made him look like a steady and chill character. The tornado? I had resembled an EF 6 storm at some points. I had spent a summer balanced precariously between what the authors of *Crucial Conversations* call "silence and violence." Would that the earth had just opened up and swallowed me whole!

I was aware that I was at one of those intersections I call "sacred and scared," a place where you know you are making a choice that can impact your life. Am I going to move in the direction of my calling, or am I going to let fear and self-loathing take me down?

What was I going to do? I had a contract for a book. I had publicized it to my friends and family. Was I seriously going to put up the white flag and throw the manuscript in the recycling bin?

Moments like this are complicated. We get caught in a loop of wanting to be better and realizing that we are still in process. I was embarrassed. I had made my mistakes in public, out loud where they had been seen and heard. Forgiving myself seemed impossible. I could not find compassion in that place.

For once, I was gentle with myself. I meditated and prayed and admitted that I was feeling I could not go on and write more about a subject I had so obviously failed at in my own life. The answer came softly: *This is about vulnerability. This is where you get to be with your own humanity.*

Being human is tedious at times. You can throw all the quotes you want at me about the importance of making mistakes, and I will be happy to nod an affirmation as long as we are talking about someone else. I am not sure what I would have done with the shame and self-loathing if I had not been writing this book. Would I have slunk away and hidden? Would I have remained defensive? Would I have tried to shrug it off as "what was right"? I don't know, but I was very aware that I had to get past myself to get on with the book.

I enjoy reading Brené Brown's work. I like her style, forthrightness, and self-disclosure. Her stories of being treated badly by people who attended her seminars or heard her speak reminded me that this was really about my willingness to be vulnerable—to make a mistake (okay, more than one), to acknowledge them, to do my best to clean up the mess, and then to show myself the love and compassion and forgiveness I would hope I could extend to someone else.

Experiencing this gave me an opportunity to look more deeply into vulnerability and to explore what is at stake when we cannot allow ourselves this gift. I literally could have stopped writing a book, a book that already had a title and a cover and a deadline! What good would that have done? It would have punished me. It would have validated negative feelings about myself. I would have borne more self-recrimination, more shame. I might have then taken those negative feelings and planted them in some other situation. More guilt. Can you see it? Can you see how not being accepting with your shortcomings can potentially create a downward spiral of no return?

I am sharing this with you because I believe these moments are pivotal—they are the ones that make us or break us. You are very plainly at the intersection of sacred and scared as you decide whether you are about to opt for self-forgiveness or hold a self-focused grudge. Can you show yourself compassion or will you beat yourself up with guilt and regret? If you allow the failure to disqualify you from your calling and your life, all the people around you will suffer as a result. The outcome of that struggle can literally be a matter of life and death.

Dr. Brown's prescription for vulnerability is to engage in life wholeheartedly. I am going to turn that around slightly and suggest that living life fully requires a courageous heart. You have to adopt a "Rocky"-style heart and sense of purpose—get pummeled, go into your corner, get new guidance and a swallow of water, and wobble back out into the center of the ring. That is literally the picture that came into my mind as I lay on my yoga mat that morning and contemplated what to do. "Get back out there!" was the answer. "Take your learning back into the center of the ring."

Reality Check

No matter how much we try to clean up our messes and make amends, there are times when there will be harsh consequences in response to our humanity. In the case of my story about the summer, a relationship of several years was at risk. That made it harder. Not only did I get to practice vulnerability but I got to have more training with nonattachment and nonpermanence as well. Regardless of what others do with our mistakes, we have to stay, we have to continue to believe in ourselves, we have to forgive and forget and move on.

We may lose people we love in the process. I wish that were not the case, but there are times when those we love cannot go where we are going. There are situations where our failures create too much pain. Maybe that teaches us the importance of staying in a relationship when we later find ourselves on the other side of the fence, when we are the ones who have been hurt or disappointed or betrayed. Perhaps part of the learning in our own most vulnerable moments is realizing the importance of staying with others in the midst of theirs.

Leaning In

There is a delicate balance in the dance of vulnerability. We have to walk fearlessly forward in spite of our own imperfections, and we also have to make room for the humanity of those around us. The moments when that perfect balance is achieved, anything is possible and miracles can happen.

Let me take you back to the story about Sam and me for a moment. I was "all in" in the potential-for-wounding game. I was emotionally exposed in at least two places. First, I admitted to the class that I was afraid of snakes. Then, I put my hand out for Sam to hold. I faced the possibility of rejection in each case. The class could have made fun of me and said "What? You are a naturalist and that's your job!" Sam could have left me hanging with a snake in one hand and an empty upturned palm in the other. But neither of those things happened. Why not?

I have my ideas about it. The kids I was teaching were, in that moment, aware of their own fears. Whatever mechanism was present in those 11-year-old heads and hearts, they were able to put themselves in my shoes. At least half of them were afraid of snakes, too. Almost every one of them was afraid of walking outdoors in the dark. I had acknowledged their fear. I had confessed mine. We were held in a perfect balance of seeing and being seen.

In the challenge course world, there are activities both high in the air and on the ground that involve "leaning in." In such situations, each partner leans into the center to support the other—the weight of one balances the weight of the other. I have done this both on the ground and 30 feet in the air. It really does not matter where you do it—when you think you are going to fall, you tend to back out … and then, of course, both people fall. It takes commitment and courage to stay in when you get afraid or lose your confidence. In the room with my group that night everyone leaned in. No one pulled out. We were all met. We were all vulnerable and all held. What that tells me is that our willingness to acknowledge not only our own vulnerability but also that of those around us is essential to everyone surviving the reality of our shared humanity.

Practicing Vulnerability Using the Second Tibetan

The heart chakra is the spiritual center impacted by the Second Tibetan. When we are faced with our own imperfections or those of another, we need a soft, open heart to be able to apply the requisite love, compassion, and forgiveness. Sam is the perfect picture. Could you not sense his soft heart? In my mind, I am picturing a large catcher's mitt where all the barbs and errors fall softly. In fact, the mitt envelops those failures in its softness. They are taken in and held, not for the purpose of being used against us later but so that they can be addressed and released—much like you would take a butterfly gently into your hands to observe it and then open your hands to release it back into the sky.

Remembering that the Sanskrit word for the heart chakra means "unbound," you can imagine what is possible in terms of vulnerability when the heart chakra is open and balanced. You can be unbound from your concerns and worries about your own imperfections. You can also be outrageously generous with the short-comings of those around you. From a balanced heart chakra you can apply love, compassion, and forgiveness, regardless of the circumstances.

I now invite you to explore the concept of vulnerability in the practice of the Second Tibetan. As you raise your body off the ground, your head goes back, and you open your heart to the heavens. In that position, you are physically vulnerable. Your hands are under you. Your throat is bared. Your chest is extended. Your most vital organs are totally exposed to the possibility of danger. You are, as they say, "throwing caution to the wind." Is that not what you do when you commit to stand in your susceptibility to be wounded, when you are willing to make your mistakes, when your failures do not set you off from your goals?

If possible, perform at least three repetitions of the Second Tibetan now. In each repetition, focus on your breathing: in as you rise and out as you return to the start position. Air is the element associated with the Second Tibetan. Feel the air expand your chest as you are lifting your hips off the ground. That expansiveness is needed when we make a mistake or have been ridiculed for taking a risk. It is too easy in such instances to let the heart shrink back and close down, to allow ourselves to retreat into smallness. As you move up into the pose, picture yourself as a beautiful hot air balloon, filling with air and rising above all that is below you. What is past is past. You are ready to journey to the next place.

After you have completed the repetitions of the Second Tibetan, rest on your back in Corpse Pose. Could this be the time to say once and for all, "I give myself the gift of being with all that I am, no matter how messy and scary"? Scan your mind and heart for any feelings of shame or ineffectiveness that might have arisen as you read the chapter and considered your own wounding and failures. In each in-breath, invite compassion and forgiveness to ride in with the air. Let that air expand your heart and chest, taking up the space that your self-wounding thoughts have inhabited. On the out-breath, visualize those thoughts or feelings moving out with the air. Continue to take deep, complete breaths until no more self-judgments remain.

If you are keeping a journey journal, I invite you to record a list of doing and being wounds that you are still carrying. Use this list as a resource for looking into your thoughts and actions during the week. If there are resistant spots that you cannot let go of, apply the practice of holding them close to your heart and acknowledging their presence: "Dear _____ (thought or feeling), I see you. I am here for you. I recognize that you are part of me. I will stay with you until you have found peace." Allow yourself time to sit with the feelings of whatever you are holding. Contemplate the learning in those feelings. What are they showing you? What is at the core of not being able to let them go? What do you need to accept about yourself to be willing to be wound-able and to move forward?

Final Thoughts

Later that night at the ranch, as my trail group and I walked up the hill to the Water Tower in the darkness created by the new moon, I felt something brush up against my leg. "Sam?" I asked out of instinct. "Yes, Flame," came the response floating up to me on the cool night air. "Good," I said, and reached down to pat his back.

We walked along together up the hill, neither of us saying much of anything. A connection had formed through our willingness to be vulnerable with each other. He had been there for me when I needed to face my fears and hold the snake; I was there for him when he needed to face his fear of the darkness—two relative strangers, one younger and one older, willing to put themselves in the hands of another. To be wound-able. To expose their fears and trust that the other person would hold that vulnerability as the sacred honor it was. It was a gift to be cherished.

CHAPTER 11

Surrender

This is fire.
Opening the third chakra, the solar plexus, the power center.
Clearing the way for walking in my Divine power and
purpose, surrendering to what is, following my guidance,
manifesting my dreams and being at peace.

They called her the Mother Tree. She was said to be almost 2,000 years old, holding her place there before the earliest settlers, perhaps even before the first men walked down from the colder climates of the north. Her lower region was bigger than a small car; her uppermost levels had been ravaged by the years and storms she had seen. She was a magnificent coastal redwood living at the edge of a boundary between a small meadow and the fog-catching redwood forest below.

The Mother Tree was the namesake of a retreat center in Northern California that 20 other "Moose" tribe members and I shared during the weeks we attended a year-long leadership program. Each time we visited the retreat center, my friends and I would sit at the Mother Tree's feet, writing and crying and pondering our learning, sometimes alone, sometimes in pairs. In the rain, darkness, and early morning fog, we sought our refuge in the midst of her enormous loving expanse. We hugged her goodbye before our departures and always wandered down immediately upon our return. She represented nurture, resilience, and wisdom—things we all desperately needed.

California coastal redwoods grow to be well over 200 feet tall. To survive in a climate that receives very little rainfall, the trees catch the fog that rolls in from the Pacific Ocean. The resulting condensation on the redwood's leaves drops to the ground to water the shallow roots. The thick pack of needles on the forest floor acts to retain the fog water that has dripped down to the ground. It is incredible to imagine that these enormous trees are sustained by the vapor of breath from the sea.

When I visited the Mother Tree, I would stand and rub my hands against her thick bark, finding solace in the feel of the thick convolutions and folds, the deep crevasses, and the wonderful earthy smell. As I became more educated about redwoods, I learned that the thickness of the bark was an evolutionary characteristic: it made her more resistant to insects and fire. The Mother Tree had obviously experienced many fires; parts of her blackened trunk at ground level had been hollowed out by the flames and heat.

The Mother Tree was not only adapted for fire, the lives of her seedling offspring were dependent on it. The small seeds of this giant mother could only find their way down to the ground and into the earth by way of the heat of the fires that would burn through the forest. The redwood's female flowers occur only at the highest branches of the tree. Once fertilized, the cones can be hundreds of feet above the ground. Fires dry the cones at the top of the tree and allow the release of the seeds. The flames also clear away the undergrowth of other plants and trees and remove the dense pack of redwood needles that cover the forest floor. This scourging opens space and allows for the seeds' germination and the upward growth of the new redwood seedlings. The remains of the burned undergrowth also return nutrients to the soil, providing nourishment for the quick growing saplings. It is a process with the mark of the hand of a master Creator.

Sitting in the shadows of the majestic Mother Tree, you could feel her willingness to stand in the midst of all that is, to allow lightning to take away her uppermost tier, to remain in the scorching heat and flames that would facilitate the release of her tiny seeds. For centuries, this amazing tree had adapted to all that Nature and man had brought to her doorstep. She was the very picture of surrendering in times of fire.

The Not-So-White Flag of Surrender

The Third Tibetan is represented by the element of fire. In this chapter, we are going to explore the way our willingness to surrender when the fires of change come to us can bring healing and growth. In the human realm, the concept of surrender is often confused with submission. Maybe you envision an army putting up the white flag and admitting defeat to its enemy. Or you recall a moment in your past when a parent or authority figure was demanding that you do something you did not want to do. Or you conjure a picture of giving up in the fight of a disease and letting it destroy your body. If you are like me, you may tense up and resist the mere thought of surrendering to someone or something.

The actual notion of surrender comes from an Old French word meaning to "give over." Historically, much has been added to that basic context. Now surrender can refer to agreeing to stop fighting, to give up control to someone else, to allow something to have influence, or to yield power or control. What I want to point out here, however, is that no matter how you define it, or under what conditions, surrender is a willful, not a passive act. Whether you put up the white flag or open your grasping hands, you are actively making a choice.

The element of choice in surrender is an important consideration when we are discussing its expression in our lives. How do we want to act following the arrival of the fires that scorch us and burn away things that are not serving us? The victim arises very quickly in those circumstances. Why do bad things always happen to me? What did I do to deserve this? We might sit and pout or get downright defiant. I was having a conversation with a client not long ago. He was telling me all the things that were happening to him and that he felt he had no options. Upon further examination, however, he admitted that he knew that he had options, but he did not like the consequences of choosing them. Not liking the consequences does not constitute a lack of options. In the case of surrendering to what is coming to us in life, we always have options. We always have a choice, both in action and in attitude.

What would having a choice and surrendering look like? What if surrendering was as simple as not being attached to the outcome of what was going on around you? What if the "giving over" was letting go of the need for things to happen in a certain way, choosing to let events unfold as they do and to put your energy into walking through the doors that open? The fires that visit us are there for our protection as well as our growth. When we kick and scream and fight against the process, we are inviting harm and perhaps even greater trauma. I want to revisit the redwoods for more insight here.

The coastal redwood population, found only in the western half of the United States, has declined dramatically over time and is now confined to a thin strip along the California coast and a small run up into Oregon. Excessive logging of the water- and insect-resistant wood led to this demise, but the lack of fires has also contributed, as the need to protect man-made buildings has meant that naturally caused fires have not been allowed to burn and do their job in maintaining the forest ecosystem. As a result, the understory and dead plant remains have accumulated on the forest floor. The cones have no heat to dry them, and the seeds that make it to the ground have no place to put down their roots. The more the forest has been protected from fire, the more catastrophic the results when fires have occurred. Too much accumulation of debris has meant too much fuel and too much destruction. The fires have burned too hot and destroyed the trees rather than just charring their resistant exteriors.

This is a powerful metaphor for our learning about surrender. While few of us would willingly choose to have significant change sweep through our lives, we do recognize the danger in letting things "pile up." How much work do we do to shift deep-seated emotional stubble when we are in the throes of falling in love or are experiencing a sweet place in our lives? Why would we want to? We want to enjoy the bliss and good fortune—as we should. And then something happens. A relationship fails or a friend dies or something else comes into your life and scorches your heart.

You are now in a position to look deeply, at both the damage in the moment and your wounding in previous times. In these periods of your life, you are standing like the Mother Tree in the midst of a fire. The undergrowth and debris are burning away around you. New seeds for your life are springing from their tiny cones. Your resilience and surrender make possible the opportunity for new growth and expansion.

'Til the Cows Come Home

One of my favorite stories in Thich Nhat Hanh's book *You are Here*, begins with the Buddha resting under a tree with his disciples after lunch. Suddenly, a man comes running up to ask the group if they have seen his cows—apparently, they have all run away, and to add to his bad luck and misery, the locusts have destroyed his sesame crop. After the man goes away, Buddha asks his disciples if they know why they are happy. He answers the question for them: "Because you have no cows."

This story helped me recognize the fact that nonattachment is possible when we understand that whatever we are hanging onto is actually a weight that prevents us from moving freely in the world. Surrender, then, actually liberates us. It allows us to unburden ourselves of the need to live in a certain way or with a certain set of circumstances.

After reading the story, I made a list of my "cows." I encourage you to make such a list as well. You can define "cows" as anything you believe to be the essence of your happiness: your job, your relationship, your money, your perfectionistic picture of who you should be, your ideas about how the world works. That last one may be the biggest cow in the herd—seeing only one way, closing yourself off to all the other possibilities that exist, you make yourself a prisoner of sorts to your beliefs about what you can and cannot have, be, or do.

The next time you find yourself resisting a cleansing fire in your life, I invite you to stop and visualize a herd of cows stampeding in your body. Take a moment to locate them. More than likely they will be centered in the middle of your chest and abdomen. Anger. Frustration. Disempowerment. Doubt. Perhaps a little sprinkling of resentment, too.

Then do that exercise we all resist doing at first (I like to believe I am not alone in this): breathe, or try to. As you become more aware of the way your body is holding these emotions, you will begin to notice that when your cows are running loose, your breathing is restricted. Your solar plexus and your diaphragm are sharing space. The tension in one creates a restriction in the other. Air does not move easily up and down from the belly to the lungs and back again. Check in with the breath. Do not force the size of the breath or its speed. Tenderly release each cow, by name, in the outbreath. Continue doing this until you feel the tension ease and your breathing return to a regular rhythm.

The Power in Surrender

If the solar plexus is the seat of personal power, why would the healing associated with the Third Tibetan be called "surrender?" That seems counterintuitive. What does surrender have to do with power? And what is the connection between surrender and doubt, the grasping behavior we identified with the Third Tibetan?

First, let us check in quickly with what power actually means. The early use of the word referred to the ability to act or do and was related to the noun version of the Old French verb *pouvoir*, to be able to. If we let go of all the other meanings of power we have developed over time, we can focus on the notion that power is the ability to do something. Power is doing. It is not that having personal power requires you to be doing something all the time, but rather that you *can* do things you want to do and are led to do. To be powerless is to be stuck, unable to do anything. Frozen. Disempowered.

How does surrendering make power possible? I would like you to think about a time recently when you were churning—too much to do, too many things to focus on, too many expectations. In the midst of this ordeal, I will wager that you had some needs and wants that were making the situation even more overwhelming. Maybe you had an agenda or a schedule that you felt compelled to meet. As you bring that situation to mind, notice what is happening in your body. Is there a tightness anywhere? How about your breathing? Is it loose and easy, or constricted? Now, consider the outcome. Did you get everything done? If not, why not? If so, what shape were you in at the end?

I can only ask you these questions because in my moments of lesser mindfulness I am the queen of what a teacher once called "whip and drive." Remember, I grew up in cattle country. So here we can bring to mind our cows again. You are trying to bring the herd in. You are yelling and snapping your whip and driving your horse and the cows hard. Got the picture? Are you exhausted yet? I used to spend most of my time either exhausted or exasperated. I was always trying to force those cows to go faster and farther than their little legs were able to go, and half the time they ended up going where they wanted to go anyway.

Now think of a time when you had a full agenda and for some reason you did not force or push. You let the situation develop naturally. You trusted the people around you. Perhaps you even gave up needing things to happen in a certain way. From a practical perspective, that is surrender. Did you accomplish your goals? If so, then you had power and you surrendered; in fact, you had power *because* you surrendered.

One meaning of surrender calls to me here: you agree to stop fighting, hiding, or resisting because you know you cannot win. In essence, you looked at the odds and realized at that point in time that continuing to fight, scratch, and scream was not in your best interest. So you let go, you detached from the outcome, but you did not give up—letting go of needing things to be a certain way and giving up are not the same thing. When you release or let go you are still moving in the direction of your guidance and your goals. You have simply stopped trying to push the rope. (Try pushing a rope sometime to drive this point home.)

How do we blend doubt into this formula with surrender and power? You will recall that doubt is one result of not being able to choose between two viable options. When we are in doubt, we are stuck, we cannot act, and our personal power is diminished. By surrendering to both options and letting the best situation emerge, we not only stop grasping and doubting but we also end up "doing." We have exhibited our power by not being frozen by an inability to act.

Taking Surrender into Your Practice of the Third Tibetan

The Third Tibetan balances the solar plexus (or third chakra). It is here that our day-to-day actions and interactions lay down their thick undergrowth of hurt and shame and doubt. Place your hand there, in the spot just below your ribs. Is it soft and pliable or rigid and taunt? Are you breathing easily into your belly or are you feeling the restriction of a too tight diaphragm? Earlier, I stated that the solar plexus is not a worrisome concept in Eastern meditative traditions; the notion that we are not in the flow of Divine order and purpose is a malady of Western culture.

The solar plexus can be the seat of our undoing. It is grasping central, the place we hold onto our stories about how things should be, how we should be. Smack dab in the middle of the body, your solar plexus rules over all that is above it and all that is below it. When the solar plexus chakra is balanced, we see a plan beyond our own, we are guided by our insight and wisdom, we experience the world as a safe place. From that perspective, we feel empowered to move forward with our guidance. We know for a fact that not only are we free to dream; we are absolutely able to manifest those dreams.

Standing in such knowing and power, you are ready when the fires come. You can surrender to them, maybe even invite them, trusting that they will burn away the things that do not serve you. You can eventually foster the intention that the fires will bring growth and life and renewal.

If you are able, move down to the floor and perform three or more repetitions of the Third Tibetan now. You will be on your knees with your toes tucked (or not) behind you. As you place your hands on your lower back, feel the immediate opening of your chest and shoulders. Remember that you want to lead into the backbend with your "wings," not your head and neck. You will inhale as you lean back. Your solar plexus will become more prominent, front and center. Visualize the chakra there spinning freely. Increase the speed of the spin with your breath. You will exhale as you return to the start position.

There is a tendency in the Third Tibetan pose to lean back and bend from the lower back and overextend the pose, to let your thighs move back with the fold rather than remain perpendicular with the floor. What a picture! Putting our back rather than our heart and solar plexus into the work of surrender.

Surrender is not about hard work, effort, or piety; it is accomplished by opening your heart and your will to the Divine plan, recognizing that greater forces than you are at work. Not being submissive and obedient, but truly trusting that the fires around you will ultimately nurture your growth and transformation. The work of the pose is to open your heart and solar plexus as they reach toward the heavens, to expand the space in your chest and abdomen. Your lower body stays in alignment, making firm contact with the ground beneath you. You can picture yourself as a mighty redwood here, standing tall over all that is around you. Release the pressure on your lower back. Let your heart do the work to lift and open your solar plexus.

When you have completed your repetitions of the Third Tibetan, lie down and rest in Child's Pose. Allow your body to take on this pose of surrender. Relax your back. Let the weight of your body fall onto your legs. Lay your arms along your sides. In this moment, connect with the reality that surrender is the path to rest

rest; struggling and grasping … struggling and grasping can be laid aside. Bring to your mind the picture of the beautiful Mother Tree waiting out the flames that licked at her trunk and branches. You know the fire will pass. Breathe deeply and completely to allow your body to continue to relax and surrender to all that is. Imagine the vapor of your rhythmic breath cooling the charred places in your heart. As you feel the soothing effect of the fog of your breath, be mindful of situations where you know you need to apply the salve of surrender. As these images come, I invite you to say, "I surrender to _____ for the purpose of my highest good." Later, record your thoughts and experiences in your journey journal.

Final Thoughts

The life cycle of a redwood depends on fire and fog, on burning and refreshing. Like the Mother Tree, you are adapted to have an intimate relationship with fire. The fires in your life may appear in many forms, such as change, illness, loss, or times of uncertainty. It is not easy to welcome the fires of changes that are brought to you. You may want to run or beg to have them extinguished. And yet, if you can surrender to their work, you will be stronger and more productive. You will step into your Divine power and purpose with more clarity and more wisdom.

CHAPTER 12

Authenticity

This is water.
Opening the belly and sacral chakra.
Creating a flow of truth and honor, authenticity,
expansiveness and creativity, acceptance and peace.

It was a glorious July morning in the Oisans valley in the southern French Alps. The sky was blue. The air still retained a bit of its early morning crispness. The light that filtered between the trees had an ethereal quality, casting glowing strips of light and shadows of darkness on the ground beneath our feet. My friend and I were off to do a climb. We wanted to get an early start start; the temperature would be rising as the morning went on. We parked the car at a little pullout off the main road and hiked over to the entrance of a small riverside activities park. Handmade signs at the entrance advertised guided rafting excursions and other water adventures.

We geared up with our packs and equipment and set off for the path near the river that led to our destination, the *via ferrata*, a route of metal and rock that would take us up the mountain face, along the river, and over to the other side. Ascending the mountain on the via ferrata, literally Italian for "iron road," is a common recreational activity in this part of the world, where climbing is as much a lifestyle as a sport. The trails of metal cable and cleats that run up and along mountains (and may include ziplines across long expanses between mountains) allow even relatively inexperienced climbers the opportunity to play on the rocks. Participants attach themselves to the line with two carabiners on a "lobster claw," a braided rope attached to the harness with two carabiners fixed to the other end. Two clips are better than one when your safety requires staying connected to the guide wire.

Our course that day was the bottom tier of a two-level via ferrata near the picturesque alpine village of St. Christophe. You enter the course from a path right at the bank of the Veneon River. It is a beautiful run—the water beneath you, the rock in front of you, the trees on the far bank. As we walked, we could see that people were already putting in rafts and kayaks, preparing to take advantage of the rapid flow of the aqua blue glacial waters coming down from the mountains above.

We clipped the carabiners of our lobster claws onto the braided gray metal line that would act as both our guide and "spotter," grabbed onto a handhold, and hoisted ourselves up onto the course. My friend was an experienced mountain climber, having trekked and climbed in India and Nepal as well as having lived and climbed in the Alps and Pyrenees for many years. I, as you deduced from the introduction, am a more reluctant climber. I love the idea of being a climber. I fantasize about standing in the one-footed yoga Tree Pose at the top of a high peak, looking down on the world below. The thought of that possibility, however, makes my stomach clench. Alas, though my heart yearns for the climb, my body believes itself more suited to life on flat, low ground.

We started along. I did pretty well for the first 10 meters or so. Large metal U-bolts had been set into the rock, providing firm footing and hand holds. A short way into the course, however, the metal cleats disappeared and I was clinging to bare rock, trying to find a place to set my boots. Looking down brought the now more distant whitewater of the river into view. I began to strain and sweat; whatever resolve and joyful anticipation I had felt in the beginning was quickly dissipating. I could feel the freeze set in. I could not move my feet. Any time I tried to get my footing, the toes of my boots simply slid away down the rock causing me to cling more tightly to the line. My legs were shaking, and I could sense the tears that were just below the surface.

In challenge-course work, most people high in a tree attached to a rope have to grapple with a fear of falling. I often suggest to my more fearful charges that they should let go, fall, and see what happens—get it over with. (Yes, ironic, I know.) I considered doing that in this situation, but it was not going to be quite that simple here. If I let go, my carabiners would follow the line, which had a lot of slack and was actually heading downhill. I would not be able to stop myself, and although I would not fall into the river below, I would have a bumpy, painful ride to the next stopping place.

In my peripheral vision, I could see a man entering the course behind us. I knew if he got on the line, it would be hard for me to go back. In addition, I was moving at a slow pace and seeing him coming made me more anxious. I did not want to feel rushed, although at that moment I was perfectly motionless.

I had to make a call: go on and do it, or throw in the towel and leave the course. The tears were breaking the surface now. I turned to my friend and said, "I need to stop." She looked at me and nodded and said, "I agree."

As we climbed down and left the course, I was devastated. I felt that I had failed. When we got to the car, I told my friend I was going to cry and then I would be okay. I did cry. In the midst of the tears, I said, "I want to be like you. I want to be able to do these things and share them with you." Translation: *I am trying so hard to be something that I am not.*

I have thought a lot about that day. There was nothing wrong with me wanting to try out the via ferrata. But my inner knowing that I was doing it to be like someone else, or to make someone else happy, was the tipoff that it was not in line with my own talents and values. That was someone else; it was not me. I love to walk and be in the mountains. I love to climb on the rocks. But I am not a mountain climber—not yet, anyway. I have bought the gear and strapped it all on. Every time I do it I feel like a fraud. Someone's little sister playing make-believe; trying to be more acceptable or to earn "brownie points." Not only is that approach to life frustrating and heart-breaking, it is also downright exhausting.

Rather than allowing me to feel more connected to the person I wanted to impress and emulate, my pursuit of "sameness" ultimately had a negative effect, both on the relationship and on me. I believed my friend's accomplishments and abilities were greater than mine, pursuits I should master to be accepted and loved. But I always felt "lesser" and "small," and I put pressure on myself to take on things that put me out beyond my growth zone and into my panic zone.

As we continue to explore the healing behaviors, authenticity is a logical successor to vulnerability and surrender. We have acknowledged our need to be "woundable" and to accept our failures, missteps, and attributes. Because we are vulnerable, we are going to be more mindful when the moments of surrender come. When we can choose not to give ourselves over to the chaos of doubt, and are more willing to accept what is, we can finally step in front of the mirror and face ourselves. We are ready to ask the question that can shift our path forever: Who am I really?

The Real Thing

"Authenticity" is a self-help buzzword these days in books and on talk shows and lecture circuits. Why is authenticity so important? What does it matter if I am showing up as "myself" or not? Why is authenticity listed in this book as a "healing" behavior?

When I was working with high school students I would often remind them that character is who you are when no one is looking. (You are going to have a question about this a few pages farther on.) As I have pondered the essence of authenticity these past months, I have determined that authenticity is who you are when everyone is looking—not when you are at home dancing alone in your underwear like Tom Cruise in *Risky Business*, but when you are out there on the stage of life in front of everyone, with all your "baggage" and talents and fears and triumphs. Who are you then?

When I did a word search about authenticity, I discovered that the original Old French form of the word authentic meant "authoritative." A parallel meaning occurred in the Greek word *authentes*, which translates as acting on one's own authority or, literally, "self-doer." The use of the word evolved into what we now think of when someone says something or someone is authentic: genuine, original, or real.

I like the Greek translation. Authenticity is acting on your own authority. This begs the question: What does authority mean? Originally, authority did not mean someone in power over someone else; it referred to a book or quotation that settled an argument. Over time, the use of the word bent toward opinion, influence, and command, but the derivation was from the Latin word *auctor*, which we would know as "author" or "leader." From all that, I am concluding that a person who is authentic is one who is acting on her own authorship, her own origins and creation. An authentic person, then, writes the course of her own life.

This was an interesting idea to play with while I was "authoring" this chapter. What does it mean to write yourself in the world? One of the first lessons I learned while writing this book was that everyone who read the chapters had a different idea about what should be in the book and how it would be presented—10 readers, 10 different ideas. At first this was overwhelming. I got defensive. But over time I figured it out: in the end, it came down to me. The content had to match my values. It had to tell my story, in my way, and with my tone. Someone else might put in more humor or shorten my stories or talk less about the Five Tibetans. I quickly learned that my job was to consider the input, let it run through my filters, then write the book that was coming from my heart.

Even as I am writing this, I am thinking what a perfect picture of authenticity that is. We have to write ourselves according to the voice of our hearts. We certainly take in the advice of trusted counsel because we know we can benefit from various perspectives. In the end, though, we must filter that information through our values and beliefs and walk boldly in the world according to our own script.

The Importance of Knowing Yourself

A pivotal concept in Stephen Cope's book *The Great Work of Your Life* is the notion that we cannot do and be everything. We are created with a particular dharma, or Divine purpose. According to Cope, assuming that we can plug in anywhere and be content is a myth. If we are going to experience the full impact of our being in the world, we will need to follow the path of our truest calling.

One of the most important parameters of following that call is to know who you are, at least enough to know when the call does not ring true. If you do not have some type of inner guidance system directing your steps, you are going to run around from here to there like our friends the pheasants, squawking and flapping and constantly in danger of flying into harm's way. As the author of your own life, you have to be able to communicate your message when the path others are trying to lead you down does not align with who you are. That is only possible if you know who you are and have the courage to stand in what you know is right for your life.

I confessed earlier that I was a tomboy growing up. I wore jeans and t-shirts before it was fashionable. I spent hours in the summer playing baseball, usually being the catcher because it was the only place the boys would let me play. I was happy to be filthy, bruised, and scabby. On Sundays, however, when I went to church, I had to transform into a "lady"—wear a dress, try to fit in with the other girls.

One of my favorite memories of those Sunday mornings was that as I got older a few of the older ladies in the church would give me "walking lessons" during the period between Sunday School and church service. The hallway in the foyer was paved with black-and-white linoleum tiles laid in a regular pattern, and one lady would start me on her end and send me down to another lady who was watching me walk. I was not to stride or swing from side to side; I was to walk the tiles as they were laid out on the floor.

I did not, and do not, resent them for it. I loved those ladies. But they were trying to get me to conform to their idea of how I, as a girl, should walk. I am sure I had a pretty rough walk—I still do, by their standards—but my walk was mine; it was a statement about who I was.

People do this to us all the time, try to change us and remodel us. We do it to other people, too. We think we know best. We feel compelled to convince someone to be or act in a certain way. When we succumb to that pressure, we take a step away from authenticity, no matter what the reason.

I find it amusing to consider that no matter how dedicated those ladies were about putting me through the paces on Sunday morning, they were not going to turn that overweight tomboy into a Barbie doll. It was not going to happen, because inside myself I knew it was not who I was. I am not sure I understood it at the time, but I did not even bother to resist them. I knew I was not going to leave the church and be that person they were trying to "help" me be.

That is my little story, but we all have them. And I would imagine most of us have bigger ones, too. If you are willing, I invite you to take a moment to think of times in your life when someone tried to "rewrite" you, to make you say or think or do or be something that you knew in your depths was not who you were. If you are keeping a journey journal, this is a good time to spend a few minutes writing about those experiences. Identifying parts of your story that someone else has tried to write over can help you elucidate aspects of your walk in the world that may not be aligned with your inner voice and guidance.

When the Stakes Are High

It's time to up the ante here. If I am going to authentically discuss the essence of authenticity, I will need to take on issues more far reaching than walking lessons at church. In that situation, no one harassed me. The little ladies were well meaning and kind. But the stakes can be much greater, the consequences of not fitting in much more dire. What do we do then?

Culturally and historically, people in minority groups have often felt coerced into "passing" as something they were not in order to have jobs, relationships, and other privileges that were held by the majority members. Skin color was changed or enhanced. Certain mannerisms and speech patterns were controlled. Marriages of convenience were made. There are numerous ways to hide who you are for the benefit of not enduring the long list of abuses that prejudice engenders. And, at what cost? What is the price paid for living in the world as something you are not?

Have you ever taken this road? Have you ever lived one life at home and another when you stepped out the door, fearing that if people knew the real you, something unfortunate would occur? I have. I "passed" as a straight person for a long time. I attended church every Sunday and sat through sermons on how people like "them" (i.e., me) were living in sin and were headed for very hot climates in the next life. I lied in court to keep my children with me. When I finally did come out, the prevailing culture of the area where I was living led me and my partner (who worked in the same school) to drive back and forth to work in separate cars every day to create the illusion that we came from different locations, and to not tell anyone who was not in our immediate circle about our relationship.

The price? I lost the trust of my children, for at least a while, as a result of saying one thing and being another. Teenagers can be fairly adamant about the fact that their parents need to be who they say they are. I was also not open at school about my own sexual orientation and relationship, even though I saw teenagers around me courageously dealing with theirs. I shied away from connecting to the kids who were more "out." It is one of my greatest regrets about that time of my life.

Ethnicity and sexual orientation are major issues from which we can create ways to address the "little stuff." But really, what is the little stuff? Thinking we are going to be judged or ostracized or harassed or kept from having the life we want for ourselves is a big deal. It does not matter whether the source of our difference is the color of our skin, our sexual orientation, our gender identity, our beliefs about God, something in our past, an addiction, or a deep-seated heart's desire.

There are no small steps to authenticity. It is a major road that we either walk or we do not. The decision to be authentic drives the process. To be honest both in our own heart and in the world is always significant work, and a big commitment. It requires an extraordinary promise to ourselves: "I will walk in the world as I was created to walk, head high, eyes and heart open."

Your Personal Flow

Water is the element of transformation for the Fourth Tibetan. Originally, I was going to choose a story about water to make that connection. But the story about my abortive attempt to climb the via ferrata does have a water element, as there was a river flowing beneath me, so I want to focus on that river now.

One of the things you can count on is that a river is going to flow as long as there is water in it. That river below me kept flowing. I walked into the park—the river flowed. I got up on the course—the river flowed. I freaked out on the course—the river flowed. I backed off and walked to the car and cried—the river flowed. A lot was happening in and around me during the time I shared with the river that day, but the river just kept on doing what it does—it flowed and filled the space that it had been given. I was happy. I was scared. I was sad. None of that caused the river to shift its character. It did not shrink, nor stop, nor change into something else.

Can you imagine the river stopping its course because of something I did? Ridiculous, is it not? The river could not be anything other than what it was. Who I was and what I was doing did not change it. There was no grasping, no chasing after or holding on.

How often do we shift our course, our actions, or our way of thinking and being for another person? How often do we try to "pass" in one way or another to please someone or avoid discomfort? If vulnerability is our "wound-ability," then authenticity is our "self-ability," our willingness and ability to stand in who we are without excuse or apology.

The summer after my via ferrata experience, I ran and jumped off a mountain with a *parapente*, a parachute. I loved every minute of it. It was me (and a stranger attached to my back) and a piece of cloth over my head floating through the air high above the same valley and the same river where I had tried making the climb the summer before. I did not feel like I was competing or trying to measure up. I ran. I picked up my legs as we neared the edge of the meadow. The mountain fell away from beneath me and I flew. That is what I want my whole life to look like.

Finding Authenticity in the Fourth Tibetan

Authenticity is an attribute generated by a balanced second, or sacral, chakra. The sacral chakra is the womb of our life. When it is open and moving we are self-confident, creative, and harmonious. We can be ourselves and be in the flow of all that is happening around us.

The Fourth Tibetan opens the sacral chakra. If there is room where you are reading, I invite you to perform three repetitions of the Fourth Tibetan now. Lie on your back. Place your hands on the sacral chakra (area below your navel) to make contact with this part of your body's energy field. You have been on a long journey from the time you were in your mother's womb. While there, you were entirely dependent on her for everything. Your very heartbeat was dictated by hers. Now, you are independent. You are able to step forward in your own way, speak with your own voice, and walk your own path. It is this sense of wholeness and completeness that I encourage you to take into your repetitions of the Fourth Tibetan now.

Begin the pose by inhaling and lifting your head and shoulders off the mat. Lift you legs straight up, as you continue to draw in the breath. Your feet are flexed, heels flexed toward the ceiling. Your upper body and your lower body move toward each other. You will exhale as you release the fold, then return your head and feet to the mat. In the next repetition, imagine that as you rise into the first part of the pose your sacral chakra is gaining energy from the movement and the tension. As you lower your legs and head, visualize that the energy is moving out into the space around you. You are creating a container for yourself with that energy. When you have completed the repetitions, visualize yourself in a cocoon of the energy of the sacral chakra for the rest of your day. You will draw confidence, creativity, and integrity from the energy. You are creating a safe place to practice being the real you.

When you have completed the Fourth Tibetan, lie back in Corpse Pose to rest. Visualize yourself as the river in the story today. Your waters are an almost turquoise blue and icy cold. The sun is shining above you. You are flowing down from the mountains into the valley below. You are passing many different places, things, and people. You never change your course. Someone is kayaking in your waters, but you do not stop flowing. Someone is fishing along your bank, but you do not slow down. Today, you are on your course, true to your path. You are generous and compassionate, and you do not give up the wonderful opportunity to be a river, to be you, regardless of the voices and actions of those around you.

After you have explored authenticity in your practice, I invite you to use your journey journal to make a list of characteristics, beliefs, and values that define the "real you." If you are following the 12-week plan, you can continue to add to the list each day during the week. Keep the list where you can view it during the day, and notice where you are most comfortable being the real you in your list. Contemplate the places you are likely not to be the real you, and journal about that as well. Take your insights into your practice each day, and intend that you will have greater clarity about the way you want to write your life in the world.

CHAPTER 13

Connection

*This is earth.
Opening the root chakra.
Creating a foundation for oneness and connection
and unity, acceptance and peace.*

It began to rain as I crested the dunes that divide Findhorn Village from the great expanse of the North Sea. While I was told before going to northwest Scotland that fall is the rainy season, I had not donned my lime green, "Lite Pak" North Face rain jacket since my first day there. It had rained a few times, mostly during the early evening or before dawn. I had enjoyed more than the normal number of sunny blue skies in that past month.

My writing book was in my backpack, so I took out the rain jacket and put it over me and the little red backpack that had carried almost everything since I had left North Carolina on a train bound for California almost a year before. With the hump on my back covered with the green rain jacket, I could only image that from a distance at that moment I might have resembled one of the mutant Ninja turtles that my children watched on television many years ago.

Once the pack and I were covered, I continued along the rocky spine of the top of the dunes. Huge chunks of red granite had been piled up to keep the dune in place in the presence of the forces of wind and water. I walked along the top, stepping over the stairs and handholds that are liberally spaced to allow visitors to move from the parking lot behind the dunes to the beach on the water's side. Someone made a comment early in my visit to Findhorn that I might want to seek out some other walks, believing I would tire of the short length of beach from Findhorn Park to Findhorn Village. It never happened. I could not imagine becoming bored with the views. The sea and sky and sand were always changing. While the land beneath my feet was somewhat the same day to day, the views I took in were constantly transforming.

When the ridgeline I was walking gave out, I took to the dunes themselves. That had been a delight since my first days on the Scottish coastline. I was not permitted to walk on or sit in the dunes in coastal North Carolina or in Northern California. Here, I could run up and down in the sand among the heather and dune grass to my heart's delight.

On this day, as the rain fell softly and steadily, I discovered how difficult it was to ascend the dunes when their sandy surfaces had absorbed water. I started up one of the taller dunes. The soft sand in the steeper part of the climb simply gave way under my feet, not allowing a foot or even a toe-hold. It was tough going, so I put my hands down to get more traction. At this point, I am certain I was a laughable sight—the huge lime-green turtle on hands and feet, crawling up the side of the dune, slipping back down a bit, moving up again, slipping down again, and continuing the pattern until it reached its destination at the top of the dune.

It pays at times to do things that make you look ridiculous. You never know what you might discover in the process. As I crested the tallest dune, I looked out across the sea and was struck by the presence of what I had begun to refer to as a "rainbow dagger." Whether it was due to the process of rainbows forming over the sea or a result of the earth's curvature that far north, rainbows in that location appear to come almost vertically from the heavens. The rainbow before me was a piece of one, disappearing up into the thick dark gray clouds roaming over the North Sea out beyond the Moray Firth. It appeared to be coming down into the sea, and the jutting of the northwest landmass was visible behind it. The rainbow was reflected in the water and made its way to me on the incoming tide.

I wanted to grab my pen and small notebook to immediately try to capture the sight in words on my paper, but the book was too small to write much, and I had left my cell phone in the room and, thus, had no camera. I had no recourse other than to sit down on the wet sand atop the dune and watch. For the next several minutes I observed, ooohed, awwed, teared up, and overflowed, as the shifting light created one rainbow form after another. Some had clear edges, others blurry ones. At one point, the rainbow receded downward until it was a fiery pink blob appearing to rest on what was likely the town of Wick at the far end of the long peninsula to my left.

As the sun continued to at once set behind me and come in and out of the clouds, the rainbow reappeared with fuzzy edges and at one point was joined by another piece of an adjacent bow. Together, they formed a large V with curved sides that reached up in front of the bank of clouds overhead. To add to the dazzling display, the sun reached a low angle and the dune grass beside me was drenched in its light. The water drops from the now-finished rain clung to and glistened on the narrow leaves of the grass, refracting back miniature photographs of the dunes and sea and sky.

I always wonder what I am meant to do in moments like this. How can I take it all in? How can I be content to walk away and leave it there? Is there a way to absorb all of that splendor into my cells and access it in dark nights or bleak mornings? All I could do was remain in my wet seat while some of the earth's most famous actors put on a show that could not be bought for any amount of money.

When I thought I could not possibly experience another perfect moment, a flock of geese came in from the east. An enormous number of them wafted over me in an undulating rendition of their characteristic V formation. I sat with my head back and watched them fly over until they had moved on into the setting sun.

Gradually, the sun found her way behind the forest and the hills along Findhorn Bay. The rainbow dissolved from the bottom up, as though being recalled by her maker into the heavens. I reluctantly arose and began my descent down the dune and over and east along the continuous line of sandy hills. The distant, but ever-present windmill guardians of Findhorn Park beckoned me back to the path that would lead me home.

As I came down a dune and into a low heather moor, I caught sight of an older gentleman to my left. He had two walking sticks and wore a flat cap. I waved and he waved back.

I called, "Did you see the rainbow?"

"Aye, yes," he replied. "Did you see the geese? So many! They were first 50 or 60, then it seemed 300."

"Yes, I saw," I said smiling. "It was a great show!"

"Yes," he answered.

I moved on, appreciating that we could each find the piece that made our own heart sing and share the joy of the other as well. Two strangers walking the beach on a Monday afternoon in Findhorn, Scotland. I went a little farther up the beach and looked back. The man was now perched on the top of a dune, having scaled it with the help of his sticks. I smiled at the sight, knowing he had seen me turn. By the time I was ready to go to the south and walk toward the windmills and ponies of Findhorn Park, he had found his way down to the wide expanse of sand created by the low tide. He was but a small, dark silhouette in the dim light of the oncoming early afternoon dusk of that perfect November day.

Perfectly Imperfect Connections

As I sat on the top of the sand dune watching the rainbows appear and disappear, I felt a moment of absolute connection with the scene in front of me and all that was around me. I was in a womb of perfection, connected to sea and sky and color, aware of the water droplets and the geese, surrendering to the moment and my inability to capture it. The world changed around me. The light shifted. The rainbows came and went and came again. The geese passed overhead. I was helpless to either stop any of it or hold it. I could only watch from my soft, damp perch, allowing each of the characters to play its part. I resigned myself to my place as the observer, the cheerleader, the one who would carry it all away in my heart.

As I write these words, I am aware that this is the last discussion of a healing behavior and the last chapter in this book. The subject is connection, a perfect ending and a perfect beginning. It represents both your last bit of work in this workshop and the fulfillment of my responsibility as the author. My work here is to draw together everything that has gone before and to leave you with a desire to delve even more deeply into your own healing and transformation.

Connection means, as you might guess, "joining together." Over time, the word evolved to have the context of relationship, but that meaning was not originally the essence of the word. Connection is the opposite of separation. We become separated, or set apart, as a result of carrying wounds, attaching and avoiding, and demanding permanence. A study of the word *separate* led me to discover that, in Latin, *"se-"* in front of another word stem denotes "without, apart, aside, on one's own." Related words include *secret*, which means "to set apart, divide, or exclude." When we disconnect, we set ourselves apart from others; we exclude them and isolate ourselves. The separation comes because we do not see that we are all connected, that a Divine thread runs through us all. We forget that we are lovingly held by forces greater than ourselves. Our minds dart about wildly; the stories take us over. Our hearts hold anger. Our doubts and fears multiply. Our grasping after things both within us and outside of us carries us away, secreted and separated. In this state, we have no hope for healing. We can only wound ourselves and others.

The first step to connection is to open ourselves to the possibility that we can survive the hurts and failures that inevitably accompany our humanity and that of those around us. Self-protection, in the long run, is self-destruction. If we hide out long enough, nursing our wounds and keeping our imperfections out of sight, we will succumb to any number of emotional and physical ailments.

Connection is like light, it only takes a little of it to break the darkness and separateness. We need but a grain of faith to take the first step toward that light. I am picturing a small child, scared by a clap of thunder, peeking out from under a blanket. Is it safe yet? It is safe enough—safe enough to take the first step, to jump out from under the blanket, run across the floor, and connect with your Source and the people around you. When you have that much courage, all the other steps will fall into place.

Connection Comes Through Nonattachment

My own journey in writing this book has involved learning the art of nonattachment, surrendering without all the kicking and screaming that usually accompany my need to let something go. Do I latch on because I believe that what I have at this moment is the best I will ever have? That is not just a limiting belief, it is a catastrophic one. While I am hanging by my fingernails to the decomposing matter of what has been, my fresh and vital life is flowing along without me. My connections break down. Like the opportunists that they are, the grasping behaviors are then free to move in and take over the show.

Relationships. Job. Money. Health. Youth. All these things shift and change over time. The land and people and stories I have shared here have given me gentle lessons about not grasping and attaching, about not holding on. The beautiful natural sights of this world change so frequently and so rapidly, grasping is futile. Having is impossible.

The stakes for learning this lesson are high. It is only through nonattachment that we are able to connect to everything—to God, to ourselves, and to our world. Nonattachment is the doorway to freedom. You cannot go "there" while you are attached "here." You cannot experience true connection while you are grabbing on for dear life to things that you cannot change. You become connect-able when you let go of all the things you are holding so tightly in your hands and open those hands to receive all the love and gifts that are around you.

I have an exercise that I do when my iron fists clamp down and tell my head that I cannot live without someone or something. I stand with my eyes closed and my hands stretched out in front of me, palms down, and say, "I am letting go of everything that does not serve me today." Sometimes I have to say that 10 times before I really believe it. When I have let go, I turn my hands over, so that my palms are facing toward the heavens, and say, "I receive all the love and joy and good gifts that are waiting for me today."

Palms open and up is a sign to your Source and everyone around you that you are ready to connect.

Connection is Our Ticket to Transformation

If you buy into the possibility that the healing behaviors offer to you an ability to connect with all that is around you, then I would like you to consider that the great leaps of transformation are also possible because of those connections. Our capacity to take the next big step in either our own personal work or in our service to the world comes as a result of our ability to be in connection.

When, as I wrote in the Introduction, I was face-down on that platform at the Lion's Leap, I was still connected—to a rope, to my friends. While I was afraid and confused and not sure how to get to the first step, I was not alone. The steps and the leap were possible because I was connected to something bigger than myself. Several pairs of strong arms would hold the tension in the rope when I fell and would let me down gently to the ground. Many helping hands would stand me upright and unclasp the ropes and set me free. The leap was possible because there was connection.

We are all in this together. Our reward for the hard work of climbing over and around in the grasping behaviors is to allow us the pure joy of our connections with the people around us. We now know we can stop the hiding. We can bring our doubts and fears into the open. We can let go of our hurts, practice forgiving ourselves and others, and step away from resentment and miserliness. We can open our hearts to love and generosity in all its forms. We can be who we are, which means we can agree with our Creator that we are perfectly made. We can celebrate our lives and our many blessings with grateful hearts. We can change. We can grow. We can leap over the barriers and fears that have held us small and uninspired. Now, transformation is not only possible, it is inevitable.

The Joy of Connection

In spite of all the wonders Mother Nature laid out for me that day on the dunes, the moments that quickly get me "leaking," as the Scots would say about tears, are those that I spent in the company of a total stranger: the older gentleman in the flat cap, me going in one direction, him in another. Each of us had our own story, our own perspective on the most amazing sight that we saw that day; both of us were connected, I am sure, by our love for the land and sea. Those few words between us created incredible joy for me at the time. I relive that pleasure each time I recall the excitement in his voice and his willingness to do the hard work of climbing with his aging legs and walking sticks to the top of that slippery dune to get a better look at the sea at the end of the day.

It was our willingness to share our lives that made those moments possible. We will probably never see each other again, but we dared to speak about what had been for each one of us moments of true joy. In our reaching out to a passing stranger, we both experienced the purest of connections—not needing, not fearing, not grasping; each of us simply sharing a piece of our hearts. For me, that is the essence of connection: joining our hearts, from a place of unconditional love, for the purpose of holding each other in the light, so that we might all walk our path in joy.

Connecting to Earth and All That Is

Earth is the element associated with the Fifth Tibetan, the solid material beneath our feet that makes our every step possible. Grounding to the earth each day is one way to insure that you will remain mindful of that connection. You can ground to the earth in many ways: eating root vegetables, walking barefoot, hugging a tree (literally). You can also ground to the earth in your meditation by visualizing that you are sending roots down from your feet or root chakra into the ground below you, deep into the heart of Mother Earth. Doing this each morning, and anytime during the day that you feel disconnected from the people and events around you, will help you reestablish a firm sense of connection and belonging.

I invite you now to move into a place where you can perform a few repetitions of the Fifth Tibetan. This time, as you do the pose, I encourage you to allow yourself to experience a sense of triumph and empowerment. You have stayed the course. You have established and maintained a personal practice. You have done the hard work of looking within. Let the Fifth Tibetan be your celebration today. Lift your body off the mat as you inhale deeply. Extend your root chakra toward the heavens. Press your head toward your heart. Listen—listen for the messages that the center of your being has for you today. Your chest is expanding as you inhale in the midst of this folding in. There is life brewing within you. You are ready for that next big leap. As you release the breath, let your arms carry your body gently back down to earth. As you arch your back and open your heart to All That Is, you are transforming your introspection into full-fledged connection with everything that is around you. It is a perfect picture of our miraculous connection to the earth below us, the sky above us, and everything in between.

As you rest in Child's Pose this last time, your arms and shoulders stretch out easily in front of you. Your lower back relaxes, fills with air, and expands as you take in each breath. You can now afford to stop and appreciate your work. Let yourself marvel at how far you have come. Each posture and each mantra has worked its magic. Now it is time to rest in this restorative pose, allowing it to reestablish the rhythm of your breathing and give your muscles and joints chance to rest. Connect to your body and your Source. In this moment, you know that you are perfectly loved, perfectly safe, perfectly protected, and perfectly perfect just the way you are.

And it is so.

Epilogue

As I put the finishing touches on this book I am not in an exotic place, such as the northern wilds of Scotland or the Alps in France; as it turns out, I am completing the text in my old hometown of Claremore, Oklahoma, the location of the coal mines in the chapter on miserliness. Again between "places," I have come to my mom's house to be able to complete the book in its contracted time frame.

It is December, a time of year when the weather is generally not yet wintry in this part of the United States; however, with the global climate being what it is these days, an ice and snow storm swept through last week, leaving area schools and many businesses shut down for several days. Now, if you are not from the American South, you may wonder how things could come to a halt over a light snowfall—no more than three inches of snow fell here, with a little sleet and ice and frigid temperatures near the 20-degree mark for five or six days. But the streets were never cleared in most places here—there is neither money nor machinery for that sort of work; I saw sand on the intersections, but no other signs that crews had been out tending the roads.

Part of my daily self-care is a long walk. While visiting here I usually cut a path through the neighborhoods to a trail that goes around the lake where my father used to take us fishing after work, and where I went as a teen to engage in things adolescents do in out-of-the-way places. (Let's leave it at that.) The snow and ice on the streets made walking treacherous, but I was determined not to miss my outdoor therapy sessions.

I ventured out the first day, bundled up in ski pants, long underwear, and heavy boots. It was about 22 degrees that day, and a brisk wind from the north created a brutal wind chill factor. My first day out was very short. There was a lot of slipping and sliding to get across the streets to be able to walk through other people's yards. As I have already confessed to my dislike of slipping and sliding, you can imagine I tried to avoid that possibility. The next day was a little better. Cars had knocked off some of the ice and snow, and a brief appearance by the sun in the afternoon had done its work to clear the pavement. I went out again, treading gingerly as I crossed an icy main street, and did three laps around the grounds of a local school.

My explorations in search of safe places to walk continued for several days. I kept trying to get to the path around the lake but always ended up turning back or taking an alternate route to circumvent the icy conditions. In fact, yesterday, a good week later, I was still picking my way past clumps of frozen snow and avoiding glassy stretches of slick ice on the sidewalks.

What came to me as I was walking yesterday was the realization that the path had gotten easier each day, and how that is such a picture of our healing and growth. The first day, I could hardly venture out without my fear of falling sending me back inside the house. The next day, I found a path out of the way of my usual route, and thereafter, the days became easier and easier, as the ice and snow cleared, the temperatures rose, and the sun shone. Today, the sunshine and temperatures above freezing will clear most of what is left. When I go out this afternoon, I will once again be able to take my old route around the lake.

I said early on that my purpose for writing this book was to assist you as you take on the work of looking deeply at your wounds and the ways they are manifesting in your life. You can imagine, I think, that writing the book has created a similar exploration for me. You have heard my many confessions. I did not write the book because I felt I had mastered all the grasping behaviors; I wrote the book because I knew I had not. I have enough knowing to understand what the obstacles are, but not yet the ability to routinely avoid them.

As I close the book, I want to encourage you to stay on the path. It is not easy to do. There will be times of failure and absolute disappointment. Even as I write this book, I feel that for every time I took my own advice in one situation, I failed to do so in three more. There were consequences—the end of a long-term relationship among them. That is a hard reality for me to swallow. I will no doubt spend time taking myself through all the principles we have explored in this workshop to regain my balance and sense of trust. As Ben says, "There is (always) 'wuk' to do."

I also want to share the bright spots with you. In the midst of writing this book, I experienced two amazing reconciliations, both with people with whom my obtuseness and their past wounding had created perfect storms for disconnection. One of those separations had lasted several years. I remained resolved to go forward, do my work, clean up my messes, and continue to believe in the power of love and forgiveness.

In each case, the fruit of my inner work was reconnection. Even my relationship with my mother shifted, as I lived with her again for the first time in 40 years in the midst of the heart-rending, hard work of finishing this book. Doing this on a daily basis was like being in a mini laboratory, looking through a microscope at both my past and my present and having to come to grips with my lack of compassion and forgiveness. (Yes, that is what caused the self-analysis in the chapter on miserliness.) Our relationship will be changed for the better as a result.

What I want to leave you with is this: life is an incredible journey. As they say in *A Course in Miracles*, it is a "journey without distance." On this journey, you are going to do your best each and every day. I believe that about you. I am beginning to believe that about me. I am finally able to believe that about my family and close relationships. You will turn back sometimes, avoid sometimes, reroute sometimes. But if you simply stay in the process, the path will clear. Your open heart and willingness to address your own stumbling blocks will allow for healing that you never imagined possible.

As you know from reading this book, I am a fan of Stephen Cope's *The Great Work of Your Life*. It is a book that I open on my portable reader when I want a boost or need perspective. I will admit that at this point in my life, though, I do not believe that finding my dharma is my greatest work. I am discovering, instead, that my greatest work is simply learning how to be gentle and compassionate with myself every day—accepting my doubts and fears, looking inward at my resentment and miserliness, wading through my confusion and lack of insight.

If I can do *that* work, then I will be fully able to live out my purpose in the world. I will understand the importance of awareness. I will be able to be vulnerable. I will more easily surrender to what is. I will then step fully into who I am with no apologies or shame and be my wonderfully created authentic self.

At that point, it is all possible. From there, I can connect to people of all colors and personalities and ideologies. From there, I can connect to my God and to the beautiful planet on which I take my every step. From a place of compassion and love for myself, I will finally be able to live out that compassion and love with every being around me. Then, and only then, will I be able to leap fully and audaciously into the life for which I have been designed. For me, at this moment, that seems to be the greatest work of my life. Thank you for being a part of that work.

Blessings
Susan

Bibliography
and References

NOTE: All word definitions were taken from *Merriam-Webster Online: Dictionary and Thesaurus* at *www.merriam-webster.com*. All discussions of word origins were supported by information from *Online Etymology Dictionary* at *www.etymonline. com*.

Brown, Brené. *Daring Greatly: How the Courage to Be Vulnerable Transforms the Way We Live, Love, Parent, and Lead*. New York, NY: Gotham. 2012.

Cope, Stephen. *The Great Work of Your Life: A Guide for the Journey to Your True Calling*. New York, NY: Bantam. 2012.

Dillard, Annie. *The Writing Life*. New York, NY: Harper Perennial. 1990.

Hạnh, Thich Nhat, and Melvin McLeod. *You Are Here: Discovering the Magic of the Present Moment*. Boston, MA: Shambhala. 2009.

Horsley, Mary. *Chakra Workout: Balancing the Chakras with Yoga*. London, UK: Gaia. 2006.

Katie, Byron, and Stephen Mitchell. *Loving What Is: Four Questions Can Change Your Life*. New York, NY: Harmony. 2002.

Kelder, Peter. *The Eye of Revelation*. Burbank, CA: The New Era Press. 1939.

_____. *Ancient Secret of the Fountain of Youth*. New York, NY: Doubleday. 1998.

Kilham, Christopher. *The Five Tibetans: Five Dynamic Exercises for Health, Energy, and Personal Power*. Rochester, VT: Healing Arts.1994.

Levine, Peter A. *Healing Trauma: A Pioneering Program for Restoring the Wisdom of Your Body*. Boulder, CO: Sounds True. 2005.

Minich, Deanna. *Chakra Foods for Optimum Health: A Guide to the Foods That Can Improve Your Energy, Inspire Creative Changes, Open Your Heart, and Heal Body, Mind, and Spirit.* San Francisco, CA: Conari. 2009.

Oldershaw, Dekyi-Lee. *www.lamponthepath.org.*

Palmer, Parker J. *Let Your Life Speak: Listening for the Voice of Vocation.* San Francisco, CA: Jossey-Bass. 2000.

Patterson, Kerry, Joseph Grenny, Al Switzler, and Ron McMillan. *Crucial Conversations.* New York, NY: McGraw-Hill. 2012.

Tolle, Eckhart. *The Power of Now: A Guide to Spiritual Enlightenment.* Novato, CA: New World Library. 1999.

Villoldo, Alberto. *Shaman, Healer, Sage: How to Heal Yourself and Others with the Energy Medicine of the Americas.* New York, NY: Harmony. 2000.

Wangyal, Tenzin, and Mark Dahlby. *Healing with Form, Energy and Light: The Five Elements in Tibetan Shamanism, Tantra, and Dzogchen.* Ithaca, NY: Snow Lion Pub. 2002.

Suggestions for Book Clubs and Groups

This is the perfect book for your group to read and discuss. Your members can follow the 12-week plan, establish their own personal practices, then come together to discuss the chapters and share their insights and learning. You will find additional resources on my website at *www.5tibetansworkshop.com* and my dedicated Facebook page, 5 Tibetans Yoga Workshop.

About the Author

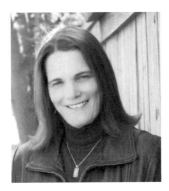

After more than 25 years as an educator and researcher in university and public school settings, Susan L. Westbrook, Ph.D., took a leap out of the mainstream to embark on a path of spiritual enlightenment and personal healing. In her journey she worked as a chef at a *gite* in France, wandered the Northern California hills teaching ecology to school children, and traveled to Scotland to become a Reiki Master/Teacher in the Usui and Karuna® traditions. Stories and lessons from those adventures have created a framework for Susan's first book, *The Five Tibetans Yoga Workshop: Tone Your Body and Transform Your Life.*

Susan is an experienced teacher and transformational coach who is passionate about helping her clients and readers heal old wounds of the heart that steal peace, joy, and abundance from life. She blends her coaching expertise, her early roots in conservative Christianity, and elements of mindfulness from the Buddhist tradition to create a unique and compassionate approach to spiritual healing able to support the paths of all seekers. Susan shares that work in her online and in-person Five Tibetans Yoga Workshops, in speaking engagements, and in sessions with private coaching clients.

Susan has two grown children, Jenny and Aaron, and is grandmother to three-year-old Ben. She currently resides in North Carolina, but is always looking for the next place to launch a new adventure.

Learn more about Susan's work and The Five Tibetans Yoga Workshop at *www.5tibetansworkshop.com* or contact her directly at *susan@mastertheleap.com.*

F I N D H O R N   P R E S S

Life-Changing Books

For a complete catalogue,
please contact:

Findhorn Press Ltd
117-121 High Street,
Forres IV36 1AB,
Scotland, UK

t +44 (0)1309 690582
f +44 (0)131 777 2711
e info@findhornpress.com

or consult our catalogue online
(with secure order facility) on
www.findhornpress.com

For information on the Findhorn Foundation:
www.findhorn.org